DISCOUNTED LIFE

Discounted Life

The Price of Global Surrogacy in India

Sharmila Rudrappa

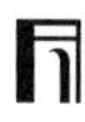

NEW YORK UNIVERSITY PRESS
New York and London

NEW YORK UNIVERSITY PRESS
New York and London
www.nyupress.org

References to Internet websites (URLs) were accurate at the time of writing. Neither the author nor New York University Press is responsible for URLs that may have expired or changed since the manuscript was prepared.

Library of Congress Cataloging-in-Publication Data
Rudrappa, Sharmila, 1966–
Discounted life : the price of global surrogacy in India / Sharmila Rudrappa.
pages cm Includes bibliographical references and index.
ISBN 978-1-4798-7452-1 (cl : alk. paper) — ISBN 978-1-4798-2532-5 (pb : alk. paper)
1. Surrogate motherhood—India. 2. Surrogate motherhood—Economic aspects—India. 3. Human reproductive technology—Social aspects—India. I. Title.
HQ759.5.R83 2016
306.874'30954—dc23 2015021426

New York University Press books are printed on acid-free paper, and their binding materials are chosen for strength and durability. We strive to use environmentally responsible suppliers and materials to the greatest extent possible in publishing our books.

Manufactured in the United States of America

10 9 8 7 6 5 4 3 2 1

Also available as an ebook

CONTENTS

ACKNOWLEDGMENTS

How easy it would be to begin and end this acknowledgment with a "Thanks, y'all!" But also how vastly inadequate in thanking people in Australia, Denmark, France, India, and the United States who've kindly held my hand, but also poked and prodded me into pushing my inquiries on global surrogacy just that much further. I'll begin by saying a heartfelt *dhanyavada-galu* to all the surrogate mothers, egg donors, and garment workers who spoke with me; I am unable to name them except through pseudonyms. I am especially grateful to the individuals I name as Roopa, Indirani, Suma, Kavita, and Salma in these pages. Without them I would never have met and interviewed 70 surrogate mothers and 31 egg donors. And, of course, Sarita too, who began this whole journey for me. I am forever grateful to all of them for their magnanimity, patience, and their labor expended in recruiting interviewees, in making lunches for us, and that overly sweet tea that emerges only from South Indian kitchens. Thank you for opening your homes and sharing your lives in far more generous ways than I could have imagined.

And the intended parents too, who shall remain unnamed. It is easy to stand outside the entire surrogacy process and cast a critical eye, but it is hard to walk in their shoes, to feel utter joy yet also trepidation in what they have begun; to love those babies more than life itself yet also question the processes unleashed. These Americans and Australians who opened their hearts continue to teach me how to listen.

To Dr. Sulochana Gunasheela whose energy, enthusiasm, and love for her work lives on. I wish I could have had this book in her hands before she left us in 2012. She was my mentor in countless big and small ways. I thank my dearest Austin friend, Jane Smith Garces. She's eagerly read multiple versions of articles and book manuscripts. And suffered through endless conversations about my troubles and tribulations in international travel, fieldwork in Bangalore, and writing. Jane has always put up with me with good humor and much love. *Muchas gracias*. I want to be just like you, Jane, when I grow up to be ninety years old.

My colleagues at UT-Austin—Ben Carrington, Donald Davis, Maya Charrad, Jennifer Glass, Sue Heinzelman, Gloria Gonzalez Lopez, Sheldon Ekland Olson, Sona Shah, Snehal Shingavi, Kamala Visweswaran, Christine Williams, Michael Young—thank you! Javier Auyero, a big thank you for reading a very early, raw version of three chapters and brainstorming over the title, with chocolate, no less! It is in these small moments that I feel like the surrogate mothers in the dormitory; that the College of Liberal Arts building is actually less and less an empty institutional space and more an engaging workplace.

I am deeply grateful to colleagues and friends outside Austin for giving me opportunities to share my work: Marcia Inhorn who invited me to be on panels with her, and to be a participant in the outstanding "Globalized Fatherhood" workshop at Yale in April 2012. In conversations with you, Marcia, and with workshop copresenters, my book grew and grew. I am grateful to other colleagues too who have been just as generous with their time and intellectual engagement. Rhacel Parreñas, Hung Cam Thai, and Rachel Silvey pulled together the "Intimate Industries" workshop at Pomona in March 2013; the workshop participants, and the three co-organizers in particular, were instrumental in helping conceptualize chapter 6, which is a much-expanded version of my presentation there and at the Yale "Globalized Fatherhood" workshop. Rachel Washburn invited me to present at the Bellarmine Forum titled "Health Now: Questions, Controversy, and the Promise of Prevention" at Loyola Marymount University in November 2012. That talk formed the nucleus of chapter 1; thank you, Rachel, for asking those critical questions on population control policies in India. Virgine Rozee convinced me to go to Mumbai for two days in November 2014, in the middle of the semester, no less, for the conference she had organized with Dr. Unisa Sayeed titled "The International Seminar on Assisted Reproductive Technologies in Northern and Southern Countries: Issues, Challenges, and Futures," at IIPS, Mumbai, October 2014. My presentation in Mumbai forms the nucleus of chapter 4.

This book wouldn't look the way it does without Barbara Katz Rothman's persuasive moral voice. Barbara pushed me to speak my mind and take a stance because my compulsion to be agreeable at *all* times can make so much of what I say appear so bland. Rick Baldoz, Adi Bharadwaj, Daphna Birenbaum-Carmeli, Wendy Chavkin, Jane Collins, Nicole Constable, Shamita Das Dasgupta, Genevieve Gilbreath, Monisha Das Gupta, Pawan Dhingra, Nina Eliasoph, Chandan Gowda, Zeynep Gurtin, Erica Haimes, Rennison Lalgee, Pei-Chia Lan, Purnima Mankekar, Michal Nahman, Judy Norsigan, Jodi O'Brien, Lisa Park, Rhacel Parreñas, Sunita Reddy at JNU, Dr. Sarojini N. of SAMA, Rachel Silvey, Arlene Stein, Banu Subramaniam, Kazuko Suzuki, Hung Cam Thai (when will your book be done, he asks me), Diego von Vocano, Mariamne Whatley, and Nancy Worcester—all your enthusiasm kept me writing.

My graduate student writing group in UT-Austin: Anima Adjepong, Travis Beaver, Kathy Hill, Monica Lugo, Michelle Mott, Emily Paine, Brandon Robinson (who straightened my life out by bringing order to the citations in this book), Vivian Shaw, Maggie Tate, Christine Wheatley, and Amina Zarrugh. The book began as a five-hundred-word salvo you prompted me to write in 2013. Those specific words are missing from this book, but the spirit that compels us to believe that another sociology is possible lives on in these pages. Other doctoral students must be thanked too; in particular I extend my gratitude to Caity Collins, David Glisch Sanchez, and Wanjira Murimi.

At the NYU Press I thank Eric Zinner for reaching out in the first place. His initial excitement was exactly what I needed to keep me going. And Ilene Kalish whose enthusiasm for this book gets me to do all sorts of revisions that I had never imagined myself doing. I might resist in the beginning, but she knows her job. She is almost always right. Thank you for your enthusiasm and patience with me, Ilene!

And of course, my salaams to Roopa Anand, Parinitha Anand, Appuanna, Teju Pratap, One Akka and Two Akka, Sumanth, Shantha, Varsha Gandhi, Vijji-akka, Umesha, my brother Vinay, Sudha Manjunatha, my parents Shymala Rudrappa and B. G. Rudrappa, and their loving, fierce siblings—Bangalore wouldn't be Bangalore without you. You are my home.

But there are other homes, as my Jeff Salamon will remind me. We have our sparkling, sweet Yashoda and our funny little Ishan. Curling up against my little ones at night as they throw their sleepy bodies around and breathe heavily through mucous-filled noses, I know they are the magic dust in my life. I look at them and begin to understand why countless intended parents from all over the world go to India for surrogacy.

Introduction

Markets in Life

The U.K.-based *Daily Mail* prints a story about surrogacy in India with the highly descriptive title, "The Designer Baby Factory: Eggs from Beautiful Eastern Europeans, Sperm from Wealthy Westerners and Embryos Implanted in Desperate Women." What follows in the article is typical of such news stories. The reporter begins:

> Above a cheap mobile phone shop in a chaotic street in north Delhi, there is a grimy apartment whose peeling walls are decorated with photographs of adoring mothers nursing their babies. The woman cooing at her child in the biggest portrait is beautiful, white and affluent-looking—in stark contrast to the flat's five residents, four of whom are pregnant, while the other is being pumped full of hormones in the hope she will soon conceive. They are all uneducated, bare-footed, dirt-poor Indian women from outlying villages—and given the emotional turmoil that awaits them, one would have thought the very last thing they would wish to do is spend their enforced nine months of confinement here gazing upon images of maternal bliss.[1]

Mapping the difficulties commissioning parents face in negotiating the red tape involved in transferring surrogated babies born in India to the United Kingdom, the article describes the surrogate mothers as miserable women who will probably be shunned by their husbands and communities. The reporter continues: "[T]hese often illiterate souls are told when they make agreements often put together by shady fixers" that all they need to do is "lie around watching TV all day, eating nutritious food they would never ordinarily be able to afford, and be dosed with vitamins and hormones."

I reproduce this article in detail not because it is the exception; instead, such a narrative is the norm in stories on surrogacy in India. These narratives invariably touch upon four themes: wealthy Westerners seeking basement bargain prices for surrogacy; designer babies made out of top-notch eggs from "beautiful" white women; clients' comeuppance as they begin to negotiate shifty infertility businesses and the legal morass in transferring babies from the East to the West; and the desperately impoverished, malnourished, oppressed, and uneducated Indian women who are somehow duped into vending their reproductive services in global intimate industries. Though these articles always speak with the requisite surrogate mother who is either a widow or whose husband's illness burdens her family with exorbitant medical bills, she almost always smiles shyly and says that no one in her extended family or village knows she is engaging in a market pregnancy.

In spite of the number of persons interviewed for a myriad of different articles and TV news reports on the phenomenon of surrogacy in India, the same story emerges, glossing over what it is that these reproductive market processes *mean* for the people who participate in them. That is, how do commissioning parents and surrogate mothers experience the marketization of pregnancy and childbirth?[2] Prior to the present historical moment women have not received wages from complete strangers for their pregnancies and childbirth; nor have parents paid total strangers to birth babies for them. Surrogacy is newsworthy precisely because it remains inconceivable to the vast majority of us.

At a basic level, surrogacy is an agreement or contract between two parties, one of whom will bear and birth a child for the other. If women are unable to carry fetuses to term, or are diagnosed with infertility, or if gay men want to have children genetically descended from them, they can enter into contracts with surrogate mothers. Traditional surrogacy where the surrogate mother uses her own eggs, though much less invasive, is far less common because she is genetically related to the fetus and exercises greater legal rights over the baby she bears. Commissioning parents use their own eggs and sperm, or if gamete "quality" is compromised, they can purchase them from egg and sperm banks in the United States, India, or elsewhere. The eggs are fertilized in petri dishes and placed in a nutritive culture for up to five days. Simultaneously, surrogate mothers are pumped with hormones to grow their uterine lining. Up to four blastocysts (called embryos, though not technically embryos at this stage) are placed in their wombs where they may grow into fetuses and full-term babies. In the case of gestational surrogacy, *two* women's bodies are stimulated with hormones in order to achieve one pregnancy; one woman's ovaries are sent into overdrive with synthetic hormones so that she hyper-ovulates and produces many eggs that can be harvested. Another woman is prepared for a pregnancy through synthetic progesterone and estrogens. This form of surrogacy, called gestational surrogacy, is most common in India and elsewhere because babies are not genetically descended from surrogate mothers, and as a result they exercise very few legal rights over the babies.

All these processes involved in surrogacy are mediated by money; commissioning parents purchase eggs or sperm and hire surrogate mothers who receive wages for their gestational services, or "rent" as some individuals will argue, who then give up a baby or two at the end of their pregnancies. These markets in reproductive services raise a whole series of questions. What does it mean to enter into a legally binding commercial contract where money is exchanged for a baby at the end of nine months? What exactly is being bought and sold? Is it a baby, or babies as the case may be? Or, is surrogacy India's emergent "rent-a-womb" industry? If pregnancy is a rental relationship between commissioning parents and surrogate mother, then what is the conception of the woman's body? What indeed is her relationship to her own body if she can "rent out" her womb? Might pregnancy be deemed a service much like other forms of intimate labor? If it is, then how do the various actors involved make sense of buying and selling such a service? How do surrogate mothers deal with giving up the babies they have borne in their bodies for nine months? What does it mean for them to receive wages for such work? How do Indian women get recruited into becoming surrogate mothers? After all, not every needy woman in India opts to become a surrogate mother. Indeed, many of us may wonder why on earth women would enter into such kinds of labor agreements—which seem to be a horrific form of alienation for most of us—where the mother nurtures life within her body yet gives it away for mere money. What drives individuals to seek out children borne by women halfway across the world? How do they negotiate the market transactions involved in buying eggs, hiring surrogate mothers, and then getting the babies "back home"? How do client parents deal with separating babies from their birth mothers, women they will probably never again see in their lives?

These are the questions that animate this book. I conducted participant observation in an infertility clinic in Bangalore for two months in 2009. I spoke with 8 heterosexual and 12 gay individuals/couples availing of infertility services in Mumbai, Anand, and Delhi in 2010–2012. All these families reside in the United States and Australia.[3] I interviewed 7 infertility specialists from Bangalore, Mumbai, and Hyderabad. I spoke with 3 lawyers who facilitate surrogacy in India and the United States. I attended a surrogacy workshop in Dallas organized by a Mumbai agency. And finally, in 2011, I interviewed 70 surrogate mothers, 31 egg donors, and 25 garment workers in Bangalore. These interviews and field research enable me to provide a far more nuanced understanding of surrogacy in India than what the media provides.

The Globalization of Reproductive Services

Up until recently, the United States has been the global leader in providing surrogacy services. Australian, Japanese, German, British, and even Indian couples facing what feels like an oppressive and despairing life sentence of infertility have come mostly to California but also to Texas in pursuit of that elusive and precious baby.[4] According to sociologist Susan Markens, fertility assistance is a $2 billion a year industry in the

United States.[5] Today, however, India has replaced the United States as the "mother destination."[6] Compared to the close to $80,000 to $100,000 price tag for a baby in the United States, surrogacy in India costs between $35,000 to $45,000. Surrogacy in India was expected to generate $2.3 billion in gross business profits annually by 2012.[7] While the Indian government had been remarkably *laissez-faire* regarding clients' sexual identifications and practices, legislation in 2012 changed that.[8] At present gay men, single individuals, and couples married for less than two years are banned from entering into surrogacy contracts. Since early 2013 the industry has been servicing only straight or heterosexual couples within India, the United States, Canada, the United Kingdom, Australia, Germany, Spain, and Japan, to name just a few countries.

Surrogacy in India is a spectacular global phenomenon. Sperm are almost always sourced from the commissioning fathers. Eggs, on the other hand, can come from various sources. The commissioning mother can use her eggs, or if her eggs are unviable, human ova can be sourced from university students in the United States. Sometimes, women from the Republic of Georgia and even South Africa are used if commissioning parents desire racial matching. Or ova can be purchased from working-class Indian women.[9] As I discuss in greater detail later, the Indian surrogate mother usually delivers the baby through a caesarian section even though all her previous children have been delivered through vaginal births. The surgeries are scheduled between the thirty-sixth and thirty-eighth weeks of pregnancy so that doctors can have complete control over the birthing process, and the arrival of the babies can be timed in accordance to the schedules of clients who may arrive from international destinations. The babies' birth certificates are prepared in the commissioning parents' names. Nowhere on this paperwork does the surrogate mother's name appear.[10]

These are indeed brave new nuclear families emerging through a multiplicity of sex cell sharing, buying, and birthing, and the movement of genetic materials and human beings across national and racial borders. Anthropologist Marcia Inhorn describes these new reproductive regimes as reproductive landscapes or "reproscapes," which entail "a distinct geography traversed by global flows of reproductive actors, technologies, body parts, money, and reproductive imaginaries."[11] Reproscapes, she notes, are new labor markets wherein Third World women assist others in meeting their reproductive goals by undergoing risky forms of hormonal stimulation and egg harvesting. Various scholars have examined the consequences of these sorts of reproductive practices by one valorized group of people for the parental activities of another group of mostly Third World women who are not just unsupported, but, more crucially, are actively discouraged from fulfilling their reproductive and parental desires.[12]

However, such global developments also have the potential to create unusual familial arrangements, deep friendships, and enduring alliances.[13] Like the women using amniocentesis and genetic testing in anthropologist Rayna Rapp's groundbreaking book, *Testing Women, Testing the Fetus*, the individuals and couples pursuing transnational surrogacy are "moral pioneers" who fall back on "local and ongoing gender, generation, class/caste relations, and religious regulation" to provide a "reassuringly continuous optic through which innovative technologies," novel situations, and unusual transnational transactions are assessed.[14] Sociologist Amrita Pande, for example, demonstrates that both surrogate mothers in India and their clients downplay the commercial aspects of surrogacy by recasting the entire transaction as gifting between sisters, or missionary work. That is, surrogate mothers cast their considerable labors as gifts to the infertile women from the West in order to make the latters' dreams of children possible. On the other hand, intended mothers from the West understand their economic transaction as rescuing or at the very least, coming to the aid of their less privileged Indian "sisters." Through payment for pregnancy, and the eventual exchange of the baby or babies as the case may be, many believe that they have assisted Indian surrogate mothers in being better mothers to their "own" children, the cash influx making available for Indian children better schools, homes, and luxury items.[15]

Through their pursuit of children genetically descended from them, commissioning parents have unleashed a whole new moral landscape that may have its origins in the morass of the market, but is nevertheless thickly interwoven with deep love, devoted parental caring, and profound familial commitment. Gay fathers, especially, are charting new norms of parenthood in Australia and the United States to a lesser extent.[16] My own research shows that if gay families are disparaged because they supposedly weaken the American or Australian national fabric, these fathers show through exemplary parental practices that they are not just as good as everyone else, but instead are stellar individuals who work incredibly hard in bringing children into this world and raising happy, well-adjusted, and lovely young people.[17]

Many intended parents I interviewed—straight or otherwise—believe they are moral pioneers because they are progenitors of a new kind of *mestizo/a*, encompassing vastly divergent genetic genealogies. The children born through surrogacy in India could emerge from sperm from biracial men, eggs from Indian Muslim donors, borne by Hindu surrogate mothers, and raised in mostly white neighborhoods in the United States or Australia. Thus, though familial genetic descendance might matter to some who come to India for surrogacy purposes, many others celebrate their children's genetic genealogies. As one of my interlocutors, Caroline, a thirty-six-year-old American who had gone to Mumbai, India, in 2008–09 with her husband for the purposes of surrogacy, laughingly and lovingly declared of her ten-month-old baby—"He's a miracle, really. Given that we're Jewish, our egg donor was Hindu, and our surrogate mother Muslim, we joke that our son is a Mu-Hin-Jew." As Caroline indicated, casting a monolithic racial identity for surrogated children is challenging under the circumstances of transnational assisted reproduction, and many parents celebrate their racially mixed children.

Surrogate mothers too, like the commissioning parents, are moral pioneers. They are often deemed immoral social agents in their communities because they bear other men's children. How could they achieve such pregnancies without sex, many people wonder.[18] Yet they are brave new workers who subject their bodies to new and relatively untested medical technologies, achieve their pregnancies through in vitro fertilizations, live out their pregnancies in surrogacy dormitories amongst strangers away from their families, birth babies, and receive wages in exchange. They are active participants in emergent intimate industries, shaping a new ethics of caring and giving a whole new meaning to the social *and* economic value of babies and motherhood.

Transnational commercial, gestational surrogacy, as I explain in this book, is undoubtedly exploitative. Yet if there is one thing I have learned since I began studying cross-border reproductive care in 2008, it is this: These global market pursuits have unleashed new ways of making multiracial families, unpacked meanings of motherhood in ways that are still confusing, and creating fraught yet extraordinary relationships between children, men, and women across the globe. This book, then, is an attempt to unpack the ambiguities in transnational surrogacy, which I broadly call a kind of *market in life*.

Markets in Life

I build the phrase "markets in life" from the concept of bioeconomies, which is understood to be a frontier technology that involves a transformation of life forms such as biofuels and hybrid crops, for the purposes of profit. This new kind of economy based on biology, that is, bioeconomy, builds from the latent value held in biological materials, which offer vast business opportunities. Sociologist Melinda Cooper notes that life itself creates surplus value, which forms the basis for profits.[19] Bioeconomies are not solely techno-scientific developments, but are political projects.[20] At the forefront of the study of bioeconomies is Australian sociologist Catherine Waldby, who in her larger oeuvre of work shows that new biological technologies reorganize human body parts and tissues to create surplus value by harvesting "marginal forms of vitality—the foetal, cadaverous, and extracted tissue, as well as bodies and body parts of the *socially* marginal" in order to "aid the intensification of vitality for other living beings."[21]

Working from the scholarship on bioeconomies I define *markets in life* as the emergent commodification of life processes that had previously not been incorporated into the market. Markets in life are organized through institutional setups, which recruit people from the social margins, bring in scientists and doctors, mobilize research and pharmaceutical products, and pull in clients from privileged sectors of societies across the world in order to sell body parts and tissue such as hair, blood, kidneys, human ova, and sperm. These markets also include experimental stem cell technologies that promise huge capital gains. Surrogacy is one kind of market in life, which comprises various elements; egg and sperm banks, infertility doctors, travel agents who facilitate international travel, medical visas, and hotels for client parents; and finally, surrogacy agencies that recruit working-class Indian women as surrogate mothers for what Barbara Katz Rothman calls "reproductive assembly lines" in order to birth babies for upper-middle-class families across the world.[22]

Most of us do not question the wages that, for example, autoworkers receive for working on cars over which they exercise no rights. And we also accept that childcare workers will provide loving caring for infants and toddlers in exchange for wages. While various forms of work have already been incorporated into the market—elder care, garment work, cleaning households, teaching—we know very little about emergent forms of wage labor. What does it mean to extend market logic to pregnancy and childbirth? Crudely paraphrasing Marx's description of capitalism in the 1800s, what newfangled forces are being unleashed by the marketization of reproduction, and what sorts of newfangled individuals are emerging, mastered by and simultaneously mastering these market processes? These individuals themselves are as much an invention of the times as the medical and technological innovations that have decoupled reproduction from sex. Embedded in an account of mothers, pregnancy, childbirth, babies, and families, this book is a story about the intrusion of the market in life processes we could not have imagined being commodified, let alone globalized.

The surrogate mothers *and* client parents who appear in this book are deeply uncertain about the kinds of reproductive market exchanges that have emerged precisely because of their pursuits. Focusing mostly on surrogate mothers in Bangalore, I argue that their ambivalence around surrogacy as both an act of gift giving and market exchange has to be located in a larger social context regarding the meanings of reproduction, the circulation of women's bodies, women's value, and women's participation in wage labor.

Working-class women's bodies have long invoked horror and hope among the Indian middle class and the nation-state. Questions of national development, economic growth indexes, and modernization anxieties have all been played out on these women's bodies, and it is within these discourses, policies, and state interventions that surrogacy must be located. It is impossible not to consider surrogacy as simply the newest form of reproductive intervention on working-class women's bodies, long preceded by population control policies. If these older policies were driven by the Indian state's anxieties around working-class women's bodies as a source of dystopic overpopulation and resultant poverty, those anxieties have now been converted to an emerging hope that these very same bodies will generate new revenue streams by being harnessed to reproductive assembly lines. Working-class women's bodies are the source for human ova and surrogacy, the cutting edge of emergent biotechnologies and medical advancement. Female sterilization and surrogacy are tied in other ways; most of the surrogate mothers I interviewed had opted for sterilization as a form of birth control. Rendered infertile for the purposes of growing their own working-class families, these women now hired themselves out to birth children for middle-class families in exchange for wages. Population control programs, I explain, are also influential in shaping the current infertility industry because many doctors who provide reproductive services today have developed invaluable skills by providing sterilization services for working-class women. The surgical sterilization of hundreds of women's bodies rehearses that other kind of reproductive intervention, that is, surrogacy. Indeed, surrogacy in India cannot be understood outside the context of population control programs. Markets in life—and surrogacy is a prime example of such a market—have to be located in the larger medicotechnical interventions that make certain bodies, specifically those of working-class Indian women, the foundation for reproductive assembly lines.

And then there are the women themselves, those whose bodies form the very raw material on which markets in life are established. What sense do these working-class women, who become egg donors and surrogate mothers, make of surrogacy? If they understood surrogacy as wage labor, then it was in comparison to their lives as workers prior to becoming surrogate mothers. Already incorporated into labor markets, specifically Bangalore's globally driven garment production, the women attempted to locate their work as surrogate mothers within that context. Was this kind of work better, and morally superior? If so, why?

Yet even as they understood surrogacy as a form of wage labor, they also simultaneously located surrogacy as a form of gift exchange by harking to another common social practice, that is, sharing babies among immediate and extended family members. For example, when Indian couples face infertility, their siblings or cousins can "gift" them a child they have birthed. The situation is analogous to an open adoption where birth parents, child, and adoptive parents all know each other. There is no formal or legal adoption process; instead, the entire process of sharing children is mediated by ongoing social relationships and obligations between the two sets of adults. The ambivalence surrogate mothers feel about surrogacy has to be located in this older, prevalent practice of sharing children. These complex negotiations that govern giving children as "gifts" have now been converted into commodity exchange among atomic, alienated agents.

The issue of market intrusion into life is not a new line of inquiry. Sociologist Arlie Hochschild, for example, has written extensively about the sorry state of "intimate life in market times."[23] Contrarily, sociologist Viviana Zelizer explains that intimacy and money have a long, entangled history. Economic transactions do not poison intimacy; instead, they characterize, nourish, or amend the various intimacies that inform social life. I take my cue from sociologists Eileen Boris and Rhacel Parreñas (2010) to map out the emergence of reproductive assembly lines in India as a form of intimate labor. Intimate labors refer to the wage labor performed by mostly migrant women employed as nannies or nurses, and the globalized trade in services such as sex tourism and call centers that deepen forms of commodification to encompass emotions and other affective states of being. Intimate labor is the paid employment involved in forging, maintaining, and managing interpersonal ties by tending to the bodily needs and wants of care recipients. Such intimate needs and wants include "sexual gratification, bodily upkeep, care for loved ones, creating and sustaining social and emotional ties, and health and hygiene maintenance."[24] Intimate industries, stated briefly, are the institutionalization of intimate labor and the unequal relationships between various actors engaged in intimate exchanges.[25] Intimate industries are globalized, and in the specific case I study—that of infertility and surrogacy—hundreds of thousands of individuals crisscross the globe in pursuit of fertility assistance, human eggs and sperm, and surrogacy services.[26]

Meeting Surrogate Mothers in Bangalore, India

I never expected to study surrogacy, especially because I arrogantly presumed I was thoroughly familiar with the topic. I had worked as a graduate student teaching assistant for Professor Nancy Worcester's renowned class, "Women and Their Bodies in Health and Disease," at the University of Wisconsin-Madison. But having faced innumerable complications in getting pregnant myself, I came to learn that my arrogance was unwarranted. There was far more to fertility than what I thought I knew. After countless miscarriages I finally gave birth to my little girl in 2007, and I returned to my childhood hometown of Bangalore with my own one-year-old toddler the following summer. I also had a research idea of sorts; I'd watched the October 2007 Oprah Show on surrogacy in the small Gujarat town of Anand, and wanted to research surrogacy in India for my next book. Perhaps I had not noticed before, but infertility clinics seemed to have mushroomed everywhere in Bangalore—Cambridge Infertility Clinic, Bangalore Assisted Conception Center, Ankur Fertility Clinic, Gunasheela IVF Center, and Fertility Clinic at the Apollo Hospitals. It is hard to imagine that a country that had historically spent so much energy controlling women's fertility with an eye on population control was now witnessing an explosion of privatized infertility assistance. Yet by 2013 there were over twenty assisted reproductive technology clinics listed in the yellow pages in Bangalore, this bustling city of 8.5 million people that is the epicenter of information technology outsourcing. These clinics have emerged in the past decade.

Not knowing where to begin my research, I resorted to old habits; I relied on family connections. My father is an Ear, Nose, and Throat surgeon and has been practicing in Bangalore since the mid-1970s. His networks among Bangalore's medical personnel are formidable. Many are either his colleagues, friends of colleagues, or students from when he taught at Bangalore Medical College early in his career. Though many infertility specialists in the city were willing to speak with me solely because I was my father's daughter, they claimed they knew no surrogate mothers. I even traveled to Hyderabad to meet with infertility specialists, but had no luck in meeting surrogate mothers. I went back to India in the summer of 2009 hoping to make some inroads. The late Dr. Sulochana Gunasheela, the most well-known gynecologist and infertility specialist in the city, tucked me under her wing, mentoring me and teaching me the basics of infertility assistance. I went to her clinic almost every single weekday for just over four hours, for two months; I interviewed her patients and sat in on her consultations. She introduced me to the doctors who worked with her, all women in their mid-thirties who cared passionately about their patients. In spite of the hectic pace of work at the Gunasheela IVF Center, these young women answered patients' questions with forbearance, worried about them endlessly, and shared with me their concerns about this or that person's anxiety regarding his or her childlessness. Yet that summer too, I met no surrogate mothers. Dr. Gunasheela worked on surrogacy cases only if her clients made all the arrangements themselves. She did not trust middlemen and surrogacy brokers, and avoided them at all costs.

All the Bangalore infertility doctors I met over the summers of 2008 and 2009 claimed they did not take on surrogacy cases because they were legally fraught; or they worried about their clients' confidentiality. One reputed infertility specialist told me she did not want a sociologist "snooping around" because she worried about her clients' confidentiality. Having given up on meeting surrogate mothers, I changed my plans to studying infertility in India, as suggested by Dr. Gunasheela. She explained that surrogacy was a last-resort measure for infertile individuals; without understanding what infertility meant to her clients I would never get a handle on surrogacy. She was right.

I returned home to Austin, Texas, with the intention of going to Bangalore the following year to begin what I'd started, that is, participant observation in infertility clinics. But my goal was interrupted. I found myself unexpectedly pregnant, and in a few short months my second child was born. I was elbow deep in changing diapers, waking up at least three times over the course of the night, and spending large chunks of the day sleeping, all the time thinking I was too old to do this the second time around. Sitting at home in Texas with a newborn baby over much of 2010, I resorted to looking up blogs of commissioning parents who went to India for surrogacy purposes. Some of these accounts of travels and travails in India were absolutely delightful; as a new mother myself and filled with wonderment at tiny toes, round cheeks, and soft-sweet baby breath, I was drawn into the world of multiple babies, car seats, toilet training, and nurseries. I cooed over the baby photos they posted on blogs. I marveled at how the surrogated babies had grown from fragile neonatal beings into dimpled, confident little toddlers. What could be a happier research topic than sweet little babies? There was love, love, and more love. And there was boundless happiness in being new parents. I contacted many commissioning parents who maintained blogs, and a few of them consented to be interviewed. I eventually interviewed twenty straight and queer couples in the United States and Australia. I am still in touch with some of these parents; I even visited three families and met their surrogated children. Some of the parents expressed their support for my research because surrogacy stories were an integral part of their own and their children's lives; they say they want to share my writing when their children come of age.

My research had so far been deeply shaped by my own reproduction routes, when out of the blue in January 2011 I received a phone call from Bangalore. It was my father. He told me that one of his patients, Sarita, a stage actress in Kannada theater in her early thirties, recruited surrogate mothers for a local Bangalore agency called Creative Options Trust for Women, or COTW. She was willing to talk with me, introduce me to her employer, Mr. Shetty, and to the surrogate mothers housed in the dormitories he owned.

COTW works with many infertility specialists in Bangalore and Chennai who rely on the Trust to recruit egg donors and surrogate mothers for their clients. The Trust also houses the mothers in dormitories, monitoring the women over the course of their contract pregnancies. Straight and gay couples arrive from all over India and throughout the world to avail of the services of COTW's surrogate mothers and Bangalore's expertise in building biological families. I arrived at COTW's surrogacy dormitory in mid-March 2011. There, tucked away among seemingly haphazard buildings that followed no code, amidst narrow alleys that barely allowed cars to pass, sat the COTW surrogacy dormitory. The nondescript building was distinguished by an unusual number of young men in their early to mid-twenties who hung around outside. There were also a plethora of motorbikes parked along the outside walls. One of them sported a sticker that read, "No one dies a virgin. In the end life fucks everyone."

At the end of my first week of daily visits to the dormitory Mr. Shetty suggested that I'd learned everything I needed to know and I was not welcome any more. The surrogate mothers were forbidden to speak with me. I was dismayed because I wanted to begin interviews in earnest but that was no longer possible. After three years of trying hard to gain access to surrogate mothers and coming so close, I was on the outside again. I was disappointed, but determined to somehow get to the networks I sensed existed. The women I'd met in the dormitory seemed to know each other very well; some were even sisters and cousins.

Fortunately, when I returned to Bangalore in the summer of 2011 Sarita introduced me to surrogate mothers Roopa, Suma, and Indirani, who then arranged interviews with other mothers either because they were recruiting agents or because their tenure at the COTW dormitory overlapped with that of the interviewees and they were now close friends. The strategies I followed to recruit interviewees closely mapped the recruitment strategies adopted in Bangalore's reproduction industry. I paid the recruiter $4 for each introduction, and I paid interviewees $20. With the exception of Roopa and Salma, the recruiters took an additional $4 from their compatriots for the "privilege" of being introduced to me. Though Mr. Shetty forbade me to come to COTW and explicitly told the surrogate mothers not to talk with me, I eventually met 70 surrogate mothers and 31 egg donors in just over four months. I also met nine women who had either sold their own babies because of poverty or had their babies stolen from them.

My payments to interviewees and recruiters mirrored Mr. Shetty's practices at COTW; he paid the recruiter up to $50 and $100 for each egg donor and surrogate mother she brought in. If the mother delivered successfully, she gave her recruiting agent a *bakshish* of up to $200. Sarita, who really started the whole research project for me, explained that this practice was justified because how else would a woman have found this "opportunity" if the agent had not brokered the deal? Former surrogate mothers were effective recruiting agents because they were best positioned to explain the processes entailed in surrogacy; but also because they were underpaid to begin with and lost more money through the requisite fees to recruiters, they needed to recuperate their earnings. Working as a recruitment agent was more remunerative in the long run than being a surrogate mother, but only by being egg donors or surrogate mothers were they able to access these other opportunities.

It made sense that Mr. Shetty paid women just $4,000 although he billed client parents close to $8,000 for the surrogate mothers' services; underpaying the women enticed them to become recruiting agents and bring fresh bodies into the industry. Moreover, recruiters were effective disciplinary agents who kept surrogate mothers in line because these were women from their neighborhoods, and they had extended kin networks.

If I had worried about not meeting an adequate number of surrogate mothers, by the end of my fieldwork I had another set of worries. I had now become the resident "expert" on surrogacy. Various acquaintances—childhood friends, my father's patients, and distant family members—asked me for advice on surrogacy services. On the other hand, the surrogate mothers asked if I could find them new clients. It was not that I had no desire to be of assistance, but I balked at the idea of getting more involved in Bangalore's reproduction industry. I distanced myself from both potential clients and workers because I had no interest or expertise in brokering surrogacy deals.

The only skills I possessed were those of a feminist labor sociologist. All I could do was explain how local labor markets in globalized intimate industries emerge, how surrogate mothers were recruited and made sense of these transnational gift/commodity exchanges, and how they negotiated positions of influence and power for themselves in progressively untenable socioeconomic conditions. Because of the ways the laws are written and the labor markets are organized, it is impossible to ignore that the surrogacy system in India is disrespectful to women, and attempts to control and disempower them. Yet it was also *not* possible to ignore what I heard again and again and again from the mothers—they maintained that their engagement in Bangalore's reproduction industry was life-affirming. Thus, my task is this: How do I make sense of the lived realities of many surrogate mothers in Bangalore where a deepening commodification of the body attended by high levels of synthetic hormonal infusions, routine transvaginal ultrasounds, and routine caesarian deliveries of babies even when women are able to deliver vaginally, are paradoxically experienced as revitalizing life events? I outline how choice, agency, and empowerment for surrogate mothers operate in an already unequal world structured by global labor markets.

The Organization of the Book

The book consists of two sections; in the first section, comprising chapters 1, 2, and 3, I describe how labor markets in surrogate mothers emerge. The first chapter tracks the *longue durée* of reproductive interventions in India, namely, population control policies followed by assisted reproductive technologies. It is within these local histories and global economies that women negotiate their everyday lives, and which form the backdrop to their decision-making processes. The second and third chapters build from my ethnographic notes and interviews with surrogate mothers. By focusing on key informants I explain how labor markets in surrogate mothers are organized. Labor markets emerge by mobilizing various agents' inherited social strategies, commonsensical ideas of how the world works, and shared gender ideologies, which in turn shape women's perceptions of economic opportunities for social mobility.

In the second section I explain how pregnancy and childbirth are incorporated into the market economy. The fourth chapter explains the context in which Bangalore's women made sense of receiving wages for pregnancy; the fact that they were already wage workers in garment sweatshops and there was already an underground exchange in babies in Bangalore shaped how women saw their own market engagements in reproduction. The fifth, sixth, and seventh chapters explore whether pregnancy in surrogacy and the resulting baby are a commodity or a gift.[27] Thinking about body parts, fluids, and gametes as a commodity or gift is not a new line of inquiry. Beginning with Titmuss's seminal *The Gift Relationship*, in which he endorses the virtues of blood donation in the United Kingdom versus the demerits of blood distribution as a commodity in the United States, the circulation of tissue fragments has been well examined.[28] What distinguishes gifts from commodities are *social relationships*; that is, commodity exchanges are transactions between individuals who have no interest in maintaining ongoing social interactions. Gift exchanges, on the other hand, are transactions where people remain in a state of reciprocal dependence on each other.[29] These three chapters, then, chart how surrogate mothers and client parents move pregnancy and the resulting babies into commodity status or deem them gifts not out of a belief in rational markets or benevolence in gifting; instead, they are engaged in negotiations over what kinds of futures—mutual reciprocity or self-contained independence—they want or do not want with each other.

Having mapped the emergence of labor markets in surrogate mothers and people's labor and consumer experiences in transnational industry, I take a different direction in the concluding chapter. I ask, What do these developments mean in the larger context of social justice? Are they a literal form of vampire capitalism where the privileged gain life by sucking the very existence out of those women who are disempowered? Or are these equitable developments that further redistribution whereby childless couples receive babies they parent for life and surrogate mothers receive wages that pull them out of precarity for life? But I jump ahead. The first chapter charts the various reproductive interventions on women's bodies in India, starting with population control and moving on to assisted reproductive technologies.

PART I

The Labor Market for Surrogate Mothers

1

Reproductive Interventions

In one of our many conversations I asked the late Dr. Sulochana Gunasheela, my mentor in Bangalore, foremost infertility specialist in the city, and feminist par excellence, why she provided infertility assistance. She replied that over the 1980s she had participated very actively in population control programs. Trained in laparoscopic sterilization at Johns Hopkins in Baltimore, she began performing sterilization surgeries on women from 1978 onward in her private ob-gyn practice and in government-sponsored "family planning" camps organized in rural areas all over the southern Indian states of Karnataka and Tamil Nadu. She said women would often ask her,"You know how to stop us from having children. But what about helping us *have* children?" That is when she began to understand what it meant for women to remain childless in a pro-natalist society such as India. As a feminist, she said, she was obligated to intervene.

With that early conversation I should have realized that the history of fertility control and fertility assistance were connected. Because of the sheer number of years of gynecological intervention and the vast number of women patients they examine, many Indian doctors such as Dr. Gunasheela have an intimate familiarity with the nuances, particularities, and idiosyncrasies of women's bodies. Their knowledge becomes intuitive because of the countless hours of work they have expended in performing pelvic examinations, assisting in birthing, conducting caesarians, and finally, sterilizing thousands of women. Dr. Gunasheela held two skill sets; one that hindered, and the other that facilitated women's fertility. These two skills, however, were meant for two different kinds of bodies.

Technologies of fertility desistance, propagated by various agencies including the Population Council and World Bank in tandem with various Third World governments, were directed at women of color, specifically at working-class women's bodies. Massive effort and funds went into population control programs in Third World countries. Yet even as the forced sterilization of the poor was taking place in India, a horrendous offshoot of population control policies was coming to a head, different sorts of developments were occurring in a laboratory at the University of Cambridge in England. In 1978, working with Dr. Steptoe at Oldham General Hospital, Dr. Edwards helped create the world's first test tube baby. If Third World poor women were having too many babies, First World infertile women were not having any babies at all. What we witness, then, are the twin development of policies directed at desisting fertility in poor women in the Third World and medicotechnical developments at assisting the fertility of privileged, mostly white women, in the First World. The technologies of desisting and assisting fertility were implemented on different bodies for very different purposes. But with transnational surrogacy both kinds of interventions are performed on the very same body. Indian working-class women's bodies are targeted for population control because they are the cause of India's "demographic deluge."[1] Yet they are simultaneously recruited as surrogate mothers and subjected to *new* medical technologies that contribute to the reproduction of upper-middle-class families in India and around the world.

In this chapter I map out the popularization of sterilization as birth control for working-class women in India, and then trace the development of commercial infertility assistance. My purpose here is to show that markets in life are shaped by *longue durée* technological interventions that make some women's bodies available for the reproductive gains of privileged others. To use anthropologist Lawrence Cohen's succinct term, these women are made bioavailable.[2] By locating surrogacy in the history of medical interventions I reveal the long-term patterns of control over working-class women's bodies that form the backdrop to India's emergence as a key reproductive hub.

Managing the "Demographic Deluge": Population Control in India

I took my digital camera with me every time I conducted interviews with surrogate mothers in Bangalore. Playing with my digital camera, they'd come upon photographs of my then seven-month-old son, and invariably ask two questions. First, was he was really *my* child? Given that they were active participants in the infertility industry, this question did not surprise me—after all, I was dark-skinned and gray-haired with a very young, light-skinned baby. He could very well be the result of "donated" eggs and surrogacy. But the second question surprised me; upon hearing that my second born was a boy my interview subjects would ask me if I had had "the operation."

Listening to my interviews all over again, I was struck by the constant references to "the operation," the English word used in Kannada to refer to female sterilization whereby women's fallopian tubes are snipped, blocked, or tied. That most of the surrogate mothers have been permanently sterilized is not remarkable, given that 37 percent of married women in India had opted for tubal ligation in 2005–06. Female sterilization is far more common in India than in any other country, including China. And it is far more common in South India than in the north.[3] While there is no exact data on how birth control choice is influenced by class, better educated and wealthier women are more likely to use the pill, IUDs, or condoms than their less privileged counterparts. In Karnataka, in 2005–06 female sterilization accounted for 90 percent of "contraception" among married women, being higher among rural women and those with lower levels of education. The median age at sterilization is 24 years. And because working-class women have fewer resources and tend to utilize state-subsidized facilities, it comes as no surprise that 87 percent of the sterilized women had their tubal ligation performed in a government facility; 49 percent of the IUD users also used a government facility.[4]

The question then is why is sterilization the most common form of birth control in India in general, and especially for southern states such as Karnataka where population levels have reached replacement rates? The answer lies in the history of population control programs. The very first state-sponsored birth control clinics were established in Karnataka, previously known as the princely state of Mysore. The erstwhile Wodeyar royal family that ruled the region of Mysore perceived fertility control as a crucial step toward modernization. Along with having an efficient irrigation system that led to the expansion of commercial sugar cane farming, rural areas around the cities of Mysore, Bangalore, and Mandya were the first regions on the Indian subcontinent to be electrified in the early 1900s.[5] And by 1930 Mysore, Bangalore, and Mandya each had a birth control clinic.[6]

However, the concerted push for intervention in reproduction came later, with Indian independence in 1947.[7] Building on anxieties regarding population size that plagued British colonial officers, India was among the first nations to emphasize population control, initiating in 1952 what was to become over the 1960s the largest state-sponsored family planning program in the world.[8] Initial family planning efforts in India were rife with conflict because various state actors held diametrically opposite views. Then Prime Minister Jawaharlal Nehru firmly believed in family planning, but Mahatma Gandhi spoke out against contraception on moral grounds because contraception relied on technological interventions that he believed harmed women. For the first decade after independence Gandhian philosophies shaped the Indian Ministry of Health's policies on birth control. However, this was soon to change; international funding agencies and foreign governments, notably the United States, worried about India's population growth. The New York-based Population Council, through the efforts of John D. Rockefeller III, with demographers, scientists, and population activists in attendance, supported Indian officials keen on population control by coordinating the efforts of various international agencies.[9] Under this international pressure Indian administrators acquiesced to population control programs, leading over the 1950s and 1960s to "increasingly coercive policies with grievous health consequences" for women.[10]

By the early 1960s various international expert committees through the Population Council, the Ford Foundation, and the World Bank began promoting intrauterine devices (IUDs) around the world, including India. Under the guidance of Dr. Guttmacher, the Population Council had popularized a spiral IUD, which could be inserted without cervical dilation and local anesthesia.[11] This spiral IUD still needed the expertise of trained physicians for insertion, and was to be inserted only after determining that the woman acceptor had no history of pelvic inflammatory disease, gynecological bleeding disorders, or congenital uterine abnormalities. Gottmacher, however, wanted minimal restrictions on the "cure for birth" because the need to control population growth was so great. J. Robert Wilson, chair of Obstetrics and Gynecology at Temple University in attendance at a conference where IUDs were discussed, agreed with Guttmacher, saying, "We must stop functioning like doctors . . . thinking about the one patient with pelvic inflammatory disease; or the one patient who might develop this, that, or some other complication."[12] Population control in Third World countries was imperative.

Indian Health Ministry administrators were reluctant to implement IUD usage without studying its effects; but Alan Guttmacher, in his varied roles as chief of obstetrics in Mt. Sinai Hospital, head of the Population Council's medical committee, and newly appointed president of Planned Parenthood–World Population, persuaded then Indian health minister, Dr. Sushila Nayar, to overrule their objections. The concerted international campaign in 1965–67 to induce 29 million women to accept IUDs had disastrous results. In some regions of India nearly half of the women with IUDs complained of prolonged bleeding, and there were documented cases of severe infections. In Bihar, for example, clinics tasked with fitting women with IUDs lacked even soap to clean their hands and sterilize instruments. Peace Corps volunteers posted there recalled that "workers would wipe bloody inserters on their saris or with a cloth after each procedure, then reuse the inserter on other patients."[13] The number of IUD acceptors fell drastically.[14] This might have seemed like a setback for population control, but by January 1966 Indira Gandhi became prime minister and the young woman leader intensified efforts toward stymieing population growth.[15]

Sripati Chandrashekar, a renowned demographer, took over as minister of Health and Family Planning. Declaring that "the greatest obstacle in the path of overall economic development is the alarming rate of population growth," Chandrashekar aimed to reduce birth rates from the prevailing rates of 41 to as low as 20–25 per 1,000 by the mid-1970s. Lyndon B. Johnson pledged $435 million in loans and credits in order to support India's ambitious population control plans.[16] In 1966 vasectomies and tubal ligations were introduced into state-sponsored birth control programs. Health workers had to achieve sterilization targets established by administrative fiat rather than ground-driven realities and regional specificities.[17] To encourage acceptors, patients were offered cash benefits to offset wage loss, transportation costs, and other incidental expenses incurred by undergoing sterilization.[18] And finally, abortions were legalized in 1971 through the Medical Termination of Pregnancy Act in a partial gesture toward population control. Yet none of this explains why female sterilization became the most common form of "birth control" in India.

Why female sterilization? A cursory examination of "family planning" in India shows that female sterilization was not necessarily the mainstay of population control programs. Rhythm methods were supplemented with condoms, but experts worried that men did not want to use condoms during sex.[19] And women could not be trusted to take fixed hormonal doses, the pill, on a regular basis. The popular notion was that these products were "birth control for the individual, not birth control for a nation."[20] If India wanted to limit its population, birth control decision making had to be removed from the hands of targeted individuals.

So why not vasectomies for men, which is a reversible procedure and is less invasive than tubal ligations performed on women? Given the ease with which vasectomies could be performed, taking a competent surgeon just ten to fifteen minutes under local anesthesia, male sterilization was initially held up as ideal because it was an easy, minimally invasive surgery that cost the state little money. Indeed, vasectomies had been popular; in 1962 more than 70 percent of the sterilizations were of men. The central state of Maharashtra, for example, conducted a five-week intensive family planning campaign in 1960 where more than 10,000 men underwent vasectomies in a camplike, carnival-like atmosphere in order to maximize group pressure.[21] The southern state of Kerala, however, pioneered mass vasectomy camps where men were given incentives of Rs.100 to opt for sterilization.[22] The first vasectomy camp set up in 1970 had 40 operating booths where 15,005 men were sterilized, which was an all-India record for the era. The second camp held in July 1971 had 50 operating booths with 100 doctors performing surgeries, which resulted in 62,913 vasectomies on men and 505 tubectomies on women.[23]

The Kerala model was quickly adopted in other parts of India, and by the early 1970s vasectomy camps, temporary mobile field hospitals in rural areas, were set up in order to maximize the number of men who could be sterilized. These camps were preceded by intensive publicity and propaganda efforts. Health officers, district development officers, elected members of village councils, local revenue officers, and teachers were urged to exert their influence on rural couples. Over 3 million vasectomies were conducted in 1970–71 alone.[24]

But vasectomies fell out of favor. In 1963, 67.3 percent of Indian couples who chose sterilization opted for vasectomies. Yet in 1980–81 that dropped to 21.4 percent, and in 1990–91 it fell to 6.2 percent.[25] By 2005–06 that figure hovered around 3 percent.[26] The low rates of vasectomies are observable in Karnataka too, where 1.2 million women underwent tubal ligations and only 14,000 men underwent vasectomies between 2006 and 2010.[27]

A large contributing factor to why vasectomies became highly unpopular was because of sterilization abuse of poor communities in India during the Emergency period between June 1975 and July 1977.[28] Faced with seemingly insurmountable economic problems, including the highest rates of inflation since independence and political problems that included charges of violating India's election laws, then Prime Minister Indira Gandhi suspended a wide range of civil rights and declared a national emergency. Opposition leaders were arrested, the press censored, and crucially for our story here, men from impoverished communities were rounded up and coercively sterilized. Spearheaded by her younger son, Sanjay Gandhi, who believed that a "demographic deluge . . . threatening to throw all socio-economic efforts off balance" was imminent, sterilization became a national priority.[29] There are a number of anecdotal accounts of villagers leaving their homes or hiding in the fields for days on end in order to escape being caught and sent to the camps. The sterilization campaign resulted in a number of deaths and the government offered compensation of up to U.S.$575 (five years' income for an unskilled agricultural laborer) for those who had died within ten days of sterilization.[30] Indira Gandhi's defeat in the March 1977 national elections is attributed to the sterilization campaigns because she lost overwhelmingly in the northern states where sterilization was pursued most aggressively.

In 1975, the year the Emergency was declared, 2.67 million people were sterilized. The following year the number reached 8.26 million individuals; 6.5 million of them between July and December 1976 alone.[31] Though women too were sterilized, over 75 percent of the targets were men.[32] In mid-1977 the Emergency measures were halted and civil rights were reinstituted. That year, a mere 948,769 sterilizations were performed; of these, 80 percent were tubal ligations on women, leading demographer Alaka Basu (1985) to observe that one of the unanticipated outcomes of the Emergency was the rapid deceleration of vasectomies and the unprecedented acceleration of female sterilization.[33] The National Population Stabilization Fund similarly notes, "[O]ver a period of time, the population programme in India has become women-centric, a sea change from the days when vasectomy or male sterilization was the dominant method."[34] Sterilization of women had become the backbone of population control programs.

Sterilization Camps for Women

From the late 1970s on the sterilization of women became a popular and preferred way to institute birth control. Urban communities were served in government hospitals, but 81 percent of the rural women who opted for sterilization received the "service" in government-run camps. The vast majority of these women had low levels of education.[35]

The southern states of Karnataka and Tamil Nadu had successfully experimented with female sterilization camps for a long time.[36] These states were effective largely because of the concerted efforts of various administrative units, and not just the health department, at the district and county levels. The well-organized Revenue Department was roped in to provide all its manpower and resources, including vehicles, to facilitate recruitment of acceptors and assist with establishing and running the sterilization camps.[37] The most commonly used spaces for sterilization camps were government-run schools in small towns, which were converted into temporary medical camps for 50–100 women. Groups of poor rural women were bused in from surrounding villages to meet with doctors and technicians who were recruited from government-run facilities and private practices in urban areas such as Bangalore. Many of these gynecologists, including Dr. Gunasheela who had a lucrative private practice, provided their services for free either because they believed in the larger national good entailed in controlling population sizes, or they believed they were providing indigent women the most effective form of birth control. To increase acceptance rates, the rural poor were given incentives in either cash or kind such as radio transistors and kitchen utensils.

The women were sterilized serially in temporary operation rooms, which were converted from classrooms for schoolchildren. Generators too were bused in to provide temporary sources of electricity needed in the makeshift operation room. After their surgeries the women rested in the camp for a couple of days in order to be observed for any complications that might develop, and then bused back home. Then the camps were disbanded and reopened up elsewhere to access a new group of rural women.[38] While acknowledging that sterilization camps are challenging in terms of meeting the standards of quality care, the Family Planning Division of the Ministry of Health and Family Welfare continues to endorse them and provides detailed information on how to set them up.[39] Such camps, which provide free sterilization to women even in these days of privatized health care, continue to be prevalent today.[40]

Most of the surrogate mothers I interviewed had opted for sterilization as a form of birth control. Their voluntary sterilization did not hinder their ability to be gestational surrogate mothers because the embryos implanted in them were prepared through in vitro fertilization with sex cells not genetically related to them. The communities of working-class women targeted by population control policies are the very same ones that provide workers for Bangalore's reproductive assembly lines. How did the anxiety that working-class women were the cause of India's demographic deluge and the nation's economic destruction get transformed into the conviction that they were making India *the* mother destination, with their reproductive labor as surrogate mothers potentially contributing $2.3 billion in annual gross business profits?

The Globalization of Assisted Reproductive Technologies

Very quickly and quietly along the heels of reproductive desistance has come another kind of intervention, namely, fertility assistance for infertile (mostly white) women in the West.[41] Whereas earlier technologies of reproduction, that is, birth control, unhinged sex from the perceived burdens of reproduction, contemporary technologies, that is, assisted reproductive technologies (ARTs), have decoupled reproduction from sex.[42] The heterosexual act of penetration is no longer necessary for pregnancy because intrauterine inseminations (IUI) and in vitro fertilizations (IVF) can lead to conception. Today, along with birth control, women's access to assisted fertilization technologies is seen as a fundamental element of their reproductive rights, which has brought pro-natalist beliefs and practices right back in through the front door.[43]

The first "test tube" baby, Louise Brown, was born in Britain on July 25, 1978, just five years after abortion was legalized in the United States. Within three years of Louise Brown's birth the first American IVF baby, Elizabeth Jordan Carr, was born. She was the fifteenth such baby in the world. Since Louise Brown's birth in 1978 medical technologies in conception and childbirth have advanced by leaps and bounds, moving very quickly from lab to consumer. The National Survey of Family Growth calculates that 15 percent of all American women reported using some kind of fertility service in their lifetime, including medical advice, tests, drugs, surgery, or other treatments.[44] Approximately one thousand women undergo IVF every week in the United States, and many of these IVFs are achieved through donated eggs.[45] In 2003, 12 percent of all in vitro fertilization procedures used donor eggs, which translated to 15,000 rounds of IVF performed on mothers who gave birth to children not related to them genetically.[46] The most recent Center for Disease Control (CDC) report notes that 176,275 assisted reproductive cycles were performed at 456 reporting clinics in the United States during the year 2012, resulting in 51,294 live births (that is, deliveries of one or more living infants) and 65,179 live born infants. Today, over 1 percent of all infants born in the United States every year are conceived using fertility assistance.[47]

Dr. Edwards and Dr. Steptoe, who pioneered the IVF procedure and were responsible for the conception of Louise Brown, jointly founded in 1980 the world's first IVF program in Bourn Hall Clinic in Cambridge in the United Kingdom to provide services and training to British and other surgeons.[48] From that small beginning thirty-five years ago, infertility clinics can be found all over the world today. According to one market study, the United States alone has 483 such clinics and 1,700 reproductive endocrinologists compete for the business opportunities afforded through infertility assistance.[49] This growth is not restricted to the United States alone; there are just over 200 infertility clinics registered with the National Association for Assisted Reproduction in India (NARI), though some sources claim there are as many as 3,000 such facilities.[50]

Dr. Edwards received the Nobel Prize in Physiology for Medicine in 2010 for his role in the development of human in vitro fertilization (IVF) therapy. His achievements, the Nobel Prize press release noted, "have made it possible to treat infertility, a medical condition afflicting a large proportion of humanity including more than 10 percent of all couples worldwide." The press release observed that 20–30 percent of the eggs that are fertilized lead to live births, and that IVF is a safe and effective therapy that gives hope to countless infertile couples around the world. Lauding Dr. Edwards's contributions to humankind, the Nobel Committee estimates that "approximately four million individuals have been born thanks to IVF."[51]

Many of those four million individuals have been born in the United States, which has been a leader in providing surrogacy services to the world.[52] By 2009 assisted reproductive technologies comprised an annual business of $4 billion in the United States.[53] Today, however, countries such as Israel and India have become infertility tourism hotspots to the extent that India has taken over the dubious distinction of being the most popular destination for the outsourcing of pregnancies.

India's first IVF baby was born just 67 days after Louise Brown, on October 3, 1978, in Calcutta through the pioneering efforts of Dr. Mukhopadhyay.[54] The second, and more widely documented, IVF birth in India occurred in 1986 in Mumbai, through the efforts of Drs. Anand Kumar and Indira Hinduja.[55] Two years later, in 1988 three other doctors in India, including Dr. Sulochana Gunasheela in Bangalore, had successfully delivered IVF babies (interviews, 2008 and 2009). With the medical expertise in place, the facilitation of global trade in services through the General Agreement in Trade in Services, the availability of cheap drugs, access to cheap labor, India's weak regulatory apparatus, and last, the commercialization of surrogacy in 2002, India has today become a major reproductive hub. Just over thirty years ago the birth of Louise Brown through in vitro fertilization was viewed as an ethically disturbing medical development. Today IVF is remarkably commonplace.

Though the separation of fertilization and pregnancy, and the resultant countless cycles of in vitro fertilizations that have been practiced on women's bodies around the world since 1978, have not completely demystified conception, they have contributed to a better understanding of the processes involved. The complexity of conception has been carefully studied, broken down into its components, specific processes parsed and subcontracted out, and finally reengineered back together into an embryo that can be grown into a baby nine months down the road. All that is needed for a potentially successful conception are mature sex cells and a woman willing to have the embryo prepared in a petri dish implanted in her. Sex cells can be purchased through sperm and egg banks, and surrogate mothers can be hired through market intermediaries.[56] The process of hyper-ovulating a "donor" to extract a large number of ova and preparing the surrogate mother's uterus for embryo implantation is fostered through a slew of synthetic hormones bearing trade names such as Clomid, Pregnyl, Lupron, and Synarel. A team of gynecologists, andrologists, embryologists, and reproductive endocrinologists mediate the entire procedure, extracting tissue, testing cells, and tracking every stage of embryonic development and implantation in order to increase the success rates of a live birth. And finally, at the end of this medically, legally, and thoroughly market-mediated process, the commissioning parents receive a baby or babies.

Sociologist Charis Thompson describes the "dynamic coordination of technical, scientific, kinship, gender, emotional, legal, political, and financial aspects of ART clinics" as the ontological choreography central to making new kinds of families.[57] Doctors, nurses, and technicians in medical labs and hospital rooms, lawyers, social workers, administrators in consular offices who give visas and passports, providers of financial services who offer loans and second mortgages on homes, sperm and egg banks, and finally, surrogacy agencies that recruit surrogate mothers all collectively synchronize their varied labors to make possible hyperovulation, ova extraction, collection of viable sperm, in vitro fertilization, implantation of embryos into medically rendered fertile women. These women are constantly monitored in order to facilitate medically mediated deliveries of babies, which are legally transferred to their intended parents.

Whereas earlier all the stages involved in infertility intervention were performed within a single nation-state, today that is no longer the case. Instead, ova can be procured, for example, from white women in the Republic of Georgia or South Africa if parents desire racially white children; sperm can be frozen and shipped from the United States; and surrogate mothers from India can all be brought together to make the much desired babies at the lowest cost possible for intended parents anywhere in the world.

Infertility Assistance as Reproductive Rights

Given the importance of parenthood for most men and women, with the birth of genetically descended children marking their parents' entry into socially recognized adulthood, infertility is currently understood as a psychologically and socially devastating medical diagnosis, with women being more stigmatized than men even when the latter are diagnosed with infertility.[58] Many authors note that infertility and human rights are inextricably linked.[59] The inability to have children is seen to compromise individuals' quality of life. Children link their parents, but especially their mothers "to the broader community, creating networks of economic, social and emotional support that expand over time. As they reach adulthood, children . . . are expected to provide and care for their parents."[60] Other than the joys children can bring to their parents' lives, having children often translates to access to elder care when parents age because developing countries have weak welfare schemes and inadequate pension funds for persons who age out of labor markets, presuming they were part of formal labor markets to begin with.

It is small wonder, then, that infertility is framed as a reproductive rights issue. Gay rights advocates in the global north also make the connection between basic human rights and gay parents' rights to birth children and raise them in queer families. Proponents of infertility treatments endorse wider availability of assisted reproductive technologies because infertility is far more prevalent in resource-poor countries, and among the poor.[61] Infertility afflicts almost 80 million women and men worldwide, with the highest prevalence among communities in sub-Saharan Africa, deemed an "infertility belt" by various population scholars.[62] Access to affordable infertility assistance is understood as a fundamental aspect of reproductive rights.[63]

When examined through such a lens, transnational surrogacy can be described as a form of cross-border reproductive care rather than reproductive tourism.[64] Individuals from Australia, England, and the United States go to India as a last resort to having children genetically related to them. Many heterosexual couples have already undergone painful and expensive infertility interventions in their own countries before turning to India; and many gay couples are unable to adopt because of legal restrictions. Germany, France, and Italy ban altruistic and commercial surrogacy. Commercial surrogacy is illegal in Australia and the United Kingdom. And gay parents may face discrimination. In the United States infertility affects families of color to a larger degree than white Americans, though the latter have greater access to assistance.[65] Women in the United States most likely to seek fertility services are non-Hispanic white, married, have incomes 300 percent above poverty level, have some form of private health care, and are college graduates.[66]

Even if ARTs exist in their own countries, individuals may find that the cost of infertility assistance closes them out of the parental market. A medical technician from San Antonio, Texas, who had twins through an Indian surrogate mother observes, "Doctors, accountants, they can afford it, but the rest of us—the teachers, the nurses, the secretaries—we can't . . . unless we go to India."[67] Individuals like her feel they are "reproductive exiles" because they have to necessarily leave home in order to access safe and affordable infertility assistance to build the families they desire.[68] Their choice to have children may be voluntary, but their decision to travel to India is made out of necessity. These reproductive travels, however, emerge within global institutional frameworks that push for the privatization of health care.

The Privatization of Health Care in India

Under the General Agreement in Trade in Services (GATS), health is now tradeable.[69] Anthropologist Andrea Wittaker notes that "WTO agreements, combined with national processes of reform, have encouraged the privatization and commercialization of health care systems across the world. . . . GATS covers the movement of consumers and providers across borders for health services" by pushing member countries to "relax their protective measures through such actions as dropping constraints required on the type and number of service providers, and limiting standards for the quality of services."[70]

Under the GATS, India is committed to four modes of health trade—services flows to and from the country's territories, namely, telemedicine and clinical trials for pharmaceutical products; the movement of people seeking services, namely, medical tourism; attracting foreign capital, including opening hospitals and research facilities; and finally, the export of medical personnel (that is, migration) to developed countries.[71] Dominated by the private sector, India's health care industry is growing at an annual rate of almost 15 percent, but public spending is even lower than before, resulting in a dilapidated network of government-run health facilities, especially in rural areas.[72] Public health care investment is among the lowest in the world, at just .09 percent of the nation's GDP.[73] Whereas healthcare was the basic right of every citizen, "it has now become a marketable commodity sold, purchased, and traded at a cost."[74]

The state is backing away from its earlier role as the key provider of health services by subsidizing private investment in health care services.[75] In order to boost foreign exchange reserves, the government actively promotes medical tourism (infertility services being a part of it) by providing financial incentives to private hospitals, reducing import tariffs for medical equipment, and expediting medical visas and joint insurance collaborations in order to facilitate medical and infertility travel.[76] And crucially, it has introduced legislation to facilitate the growth of privatized infertility services. Commercial surrogacy was legalized in 2002, and ever since there have been ongoing efforts to pass the Assisted Reproductive Technology Regulation Bill (2008, 2010, and 2013 versions) to smoothen commercial transactions in reproduction.

Fertility assistance, for which India is now globally renowned, is privatized and expensive. It is not meant for the 8 to 10 million Indian couples estimated to be childless.[77] These indigent, infertile individuals are true exiles from the world of assisted reproduction, which is only available to those like the medical technician from San Antonio, Texas, with relative class privilege.[78] According to a study conducted by the Confederation of Indian Industry (CII), infertility services is a $2 billion industry. The study estimates that in 2012 nearly 10,000 foreign clients visited India for reproductive services; of these, nearly 30 percent were either single or queer-identified.[79]

At present, however, single and gay parents are no longer allowed to visit India for surrogacy purposes, ostensibly to protect the surrogate mother's rights. The Delhi-based SAMA Resource Group for Women and Health, among a host of other social commentators, notes that the current Assisted Reproductive Technology (Regulation) Bill, 2013, is more inequitable than before. The clause against gay parents in the draft bill "is discriminatory, baseless, and a violation of rights to equality, freedom, and reproduction," claims SAMA.[80] Moreover, SAMA has repeatedly criticized the draft bill as being overly market friendly to the detriment of surrogate mother's rights.

The main purpose of India's proposed Assisted Reproductive Technology Bill is to streamline business practices by providing coherent definitions of parentage, delineate the roles of the various actors involved, and allocate regulatory responsibility among different government agencies.[81] The assumption is that clear guidelines will allow all participants to enter into market transactions with a coherent understanding of the processes, meanings, and terms governing trade in reproduction. Rules that regulate surrogacy in India endorse markets as the best way to provide reproductive services because markets ostensibly protect individual rights. People wanting children genetically descended from them are able to achieve their parental dreams by paying women what is perceived to be a fair wage for their reproductive services. Everyone allegedly gains through such an exchange because all are free to buy or sell their labor and are free to use their wages, that is, consume as they choose.

There is little recognition among Indian legislators that transnational surrogacy is a classic case of stratified reproduction that results in unequal transactions because these are exchanges between already unequal social actors.[82] Even when individual clients are genuinely good human beings, feel deep gratitude, and adequately express their everlasting appreciation to their surrogate mothers they cannot overcome the structural inequalities that exist between them. The physical and emotional health costs of creating and birthing babies are differentially borne by relatively privileged clients and relatively disempowered workers in reproductive markets. The global economic and political hierarchy of nations, which shapes persons' vastly unequal access to resources, has consequences for the way First World clients and Third World workers experience parenthood. Surrogacy agencies and infertility doctors are far more solicitous, attentive, caring, and alert towards client parents' physical and emotional needs than those of the surrogate mothers. The latter's mother-work in their own families, their rights to bodily integrity, to refuse or accept medical interventions, and their feelings about pregnancy and choice in childbirth are more or less disregarded.[83]

Yet the question remains, If they are treated so badly, why do working-class Indian women choose to participate in surrogacy? Indicating the number of women wanting to be employed, a doctor from Mumbai remarked in a Dallas surrogacy workshop I attended, "Any time you decide is right for you, we can work with you. At any given time we have at least two or three women ready to be surrogates."[84]

Recruiting Surrogate Mothers

My premise is that it is not enough for jobs, such as cleaning homes, child care, nursing, or teaching to exist. Instead, people must want to *jump* into these jobs. Crushing economic circumstances, including disappearing socially provided health care, can certainly push people into selling their labor but they also need to be aware of new employment opportunities such as surrogacy, and they need to perceive such new employment as suitable work. As sociologist Fred Block perceptively notes, an "individual's capacity to work is not innate; it is socially created and sustained."[85] Taking my lead from labor market theorists, I posit that labor markets do not arise out of thin air but are social and political constructions that involve cultural perceptions of what is or is not work, and the state's active involvement in keeping labor markets open. Labor markets entail the incorporation of individual workers into labor flows and their allocation to specific jobs. In addition, to extract labor effort, workers must be controlled; and finally, the labor force must be reproduced in order for an industry to be sustained.[86]

The commonplace understanding is that surrogacy is tied to poverty; that is, women who are desperately poor become surrogate mothers because of the money they receive. Yet popular media sources that propagate this notion themselves provide alternative perspectives. For example, in an article on surrogacy in the women's magazine *Marie Claire* a central protagonist is Rubina Mondal, a former bank clerk. She appears again in a subsequent article in the U.K.'s *Mail Online*, this time as the manager of a dormitory that houses ten surrogate mothers working for Dr. Nayna Patel in Anand, Gujarat. Similarly, the Canadian women's magazine *Chatelaine* features Rekha, who says that surrogacy is far more lucrative than her old job in a pharmaceutical lab.[87]

Surrogacy agencies do *not* recruit poverty-stricken women. Many of these impoverished women's bodies and physical demeanor do not meet the market requirements for an ideal reproductive worker. Their health may be compromised because of years of living in poverty; they may be malnutritioned and underweight. They may have poor dental health. And because they lack permanent housing and adequate supplies of potable water, they may lack the prerequisite ideals of bodily hygiene embodied in clean clothing. These women may not wear sandals on their feet. And finally, they might not adorn themselves with the gold earrings and necklaces sported almost universally by South Indian women, and perhaps their hair is not neatly oiled, combed, and coiffed with jasmine flowers as preferred by women in the region. Such indigent women are automatically written out of reproductive assembly lines; instead, recruiters, doctors, and clients prefer women who come from solid working-class backgrounds who live in some permanent housing of sorts, have access to potable water to bathe daily and wash their clothes often, and can afford to eat regular, healthy meals.

Even among such women, not all are suitable "raw" material for surrogacy. Agencies seek women in prime reproductive age between their twenties and thirties. As per Indian regulations, they must be married (or separated/divorced/widowed), and must necessarily have children. The logic behind this stipulation is that pregnancy and childbirth cannot be comprehended intellectually or imaginatively. Only a woman who has undergone childbirth can be truly ready for the labor experience for which she has contracted. In addition, the belief is that a woman who has a child of her own is less likely to get emotionally attached to the surrogated child. Ideal candidates, according to infertility specialists, are those who have sympathetic husbands and access to household help through extended families. Moreover, their families should have adequate financial resources to support their children without making demands on the surrogate mother during her labor term at the surrogacy dormitory. Women are also screened to eliminate individuals who might not be able to emotionally separate from the fetus they carry for nine months, or might exhibit "post-contractual opportunistic behavior."[88] That is, they might make demands on the contracting parents once pregnant and therefore be undesirable workers.

Despite these stipulations, there are enough desirable workers in India that it has become a major global reproductive hub. Skilled doctors are available, many of whom have honed their skills through reproductive interventions on thousands of women's bodies. But crucially, there are hundreds of working-class women who hire out as mothers, who are *willing* participants in the production process, which entails their compliance to staying in surrogacy dormitories, invasive medical technologies, and finally, to giving up the babies they birth often through caesarian surgeries. Building from my ethnography in Bangalore, in the next two chapters I convey how labor markets in surrogate mothers emerge. Women sign up because they have prior social relationships with their recruiting agents. That is, recruiters convert their social networks into market networks. Persuasion, inducement, coercion, fear, love, trust, and all those nonmarket emotions that form the contours of social relationships also shape reproductive labor markets. Labor markets in surrogate mothers are efficient because of nonmarket, social relationships. The market and nonmarket were so tightly intertwined that attempts to untangle them became mere theoretical exercises rather than empirical realities.

2

Converting Social Networks into Labor Markets

Sarita: Recruitment by Creating Fear and Anxiety

If not for Sarita I would not have met the surrogate mothers and egg donors I did in Bangalore. Frequently sick with allergies and nasal infections, she was my physician father's patient. I would either go over to meet her at her parents' home or Sarita would meet me at my father's hospital where she was scheduled to get yet another round of antibiotics. She could not afford to fall sick because she was a stage actor in Kannada plays. "Stage artistes," she said to me, "we are nothing without our voices. If I don't sing or dance, the stove cannot be turned on in our home that day. I have to go and earn money every single day." Apparently my father did not want to prescribe her these antibiotics but Sarita would show up and insist on receiving medication. She said to me, "Your father's medicines have worked wonders to keep me working. I just need to see his face and I feel better. He is a very good man. You must know you are very lucky to have a father like him. This is your *punya*."[1] At these times, when she simultaneously sang my father's praises and enviously pointed to my privileged life, I'd embarrassedly attempt to construct an appropriate reply.

Sarita had a difficult life. Malyalees, her parents were born and raised in Bangalore. Sarita had never been to Kerala herself, and would not identify her caste. She was in her early thirties and lived with her parents and seven-year-old daughter. Her husband had disappeared on her; she had not seen him in years. He made occasional phone calls but never sent money. Sarita's two sisters' children went to good private schools but she was unable to do that for her own child because she supported her parents. Both were chronically sick; her father had prostate cancer and she paid for his medical bills. Yet he constantly made derogatory remarks about her and her sexual mores. Sarita often wished her mother would die because there would be one less person to provide for. Caring for her mother had been challenging, especially because her mother had had recurrent cancer since Sarita was eleven years old. First it was uterine cancer and the mother had her uterus removed. Then she had breast cancer for which she had a mastectomy. And now she had leukemia. As she narrated her mother's various illnesses, Sarita began to cry. She said, "What to do? This is my fate. This is what god has deemed for me and so it shall be. I do everything for that woman. On time. Always on time." Sarita had been an attractive child and her mother had pushed her into becoming a child actor in the Kannada television industry to earn money for the family because their medical bills were so large. But if her mother died, Sarita asked rhetorically, who would help with her daughter? She would never do to her own daughter what her mother had done to her, Sarita declared. She'd arrange her daughter's marriage to a good man by the time she turned eighteen. She wanted her married into a respectable household and not struggle like she did, being sexually harassed and propositioned at every turn.

I would eventually learn that Sarita's stories were inconsistent. She had sold her eggs two or three times. Because she needed her absent husband's permission to do so, her brother-in-law had signed legal papers to assist her. However, she also told me that no one in her family knew she had sold her eggs; instead, her "boyfriend" had posed as her husband to sign the papers. She told me she earned $500 each time she donated her eggs. But at other times she said she earned $600—more than what others made—because she was attractive and well-educated. There were many such stories.[2]

Though she had initially told me she was an actor in the Kannada theater, Sarita said she rarely performed on stage. Instead, firms or NGOs might invite her and a group of artistes to stage a private performance for which they'd collectively receive approximately $500. Because of her experience as a performer she ran her own dance school, and was the sole teacher there. Another time she introduced me to her daughter's school principal as someone who had come from America for just two weeks to see her dance performance. Apparently I was a talent scout of sorts and was ready to fly her overseas. Sarita later apologized, saying she did not want the school principal to know she worked in a surrogacy agency. One time, when I stopped by her house her "absent" husband had mysteriously reappeared from Dubai and was staying with the family. He did not seem estranged, and the entire family treated him like he was an integral part of the household. Although Sarita's stories were reliably erratic I was able to piece together that she earned between $120 and $450 per month, and though not poor, because her parents owned their home in the city and did not pay rent or mortgage, they led economically precarious lives. In her early thirties, Sarita knew her ability to bring in money would shrink as she aged, so she tried to maximize her earnings through the networks she built. She carefully nurtured the most important nodes on her numerous networks.

Mr. Shetty was one such node with vast networks in Bangalore and surrounding towns. Because Mr. Shetty was reputed to be a social worker and had registered Creative Options Trust for Women as a "not-for-profit" organization, Sarita had first met with him to finance her dance school's "Annual Day." From that first meeting onward he funded most of her school's events. Eventually Sarita began recruiting egg donors and surrogate mothers for him. "It's easy, *akka*," she said. "All I do is stand outside in the mornings with my cup of coffee when garment workers walk by to catch their bus to work. I call out greetings to them, and little by little we get to know each other." Over time she'd gauged who needed money and recruited them to donate their ova or become surrogate mothers.

Unlike most others who carried just one, Sarita carried three cell phones in her purse at all times. Two were hers for personal calls; she had purchased a new cell phone and didn't want to give up the old one because it had sentimental value, she said, so she held onto both. Her third cell phone was given to her by Mr. Shetty, who provided all his COTW workers with phones so he could contact them at a moment's notice, but more importantly so he could track all their communications. Sarita had devised her own filing system through these phones; she kept her networks separate by giving different sets of people one or the other phone number. Sarita went by a different name on each of the three phones. My father introduced me to her as Swetha and her family too called her by that name. On the COTW cell phone she was Sarita. On the third line, which she used less frequently but which she answered a few times when we met, she went by Dolly.

One morning I was scheduled to meet Sarita at my father's hospital where she was receiving her prescription of antibiotics. From there we were supposed to head out to her home to meet a group of surrogate mothers. When I walked in, Sarita was talking agitatedly on one of her three phones. Upon seeing me she quickly ended her distressed conversation. She tearfully wiped her eyes, saying she had just hung up on her mother who said Mr. Shetty had called the house once again and demanded that she repay the loan he'd given her. Sarita's troubles had begun the previous day when she text messaged the receptionist at COTW to ask for recruiter Jyothi's telephone number. This was obviously to assist me, she said, but instead she lied to the receptionist that she wanted to talk with Jyothi about the gym she was starting. Mr. Shetty had intercepted her text message and was furious because he suspected Sarita had continued to work with me in open defiance of his explicit orders. He came by her home and swore at her in front of her parents and child, using all sorts of vulgar language. She began to sob uncontrollably, tears, snot, and saliva intermingling freely on her face as she recounted that she had borrowed $1,000 from him when she'd first begun work there. Mr. Shetty demanded that she pay him back $200 immediately or have sex with him to buy herself time.

She told me that a month after starting to work there Mr. Shetty, who was legally married, began stroking her arms and demanding sex from her. His other girlfriend too, who worked as the dormitory manager and lived on the COTW premises with him, harassed Sarita. She often asked, "What will you lose? It's just one night, after all." She began sobbing when she explained this was why she had left his employment, but she returned because she needed money to support her family. I was disconcerted. Sarita had initially told me she left COTW because Mr. Shetty's girlfriend was jealous and had been very rude to her. This was a plausible story because Sarita was an attractive and vivacious woman. Moreover, some of the surrogate mothers had recounted their own difficult dealings with the COTW dormitory manager, Mr. Shetty's lover. His wife was wonderful, they had said; instead, he had now hooked up with this woman who made their dorm life miserable. His girlfriend was to play a central role in Mr. Shetty's legal travails. He married her too, and his first and only legal wife filed a case of bigamy against him in the summer of 2011. These legal troubles had led to investigations into his business dealings.

Over the course of its investigations, the Bruhat Bangalore Mahanagara Palike (BBMP), which is the state administrative body responsible for the metropolitan area's civic and infrastructural assets, declared that Mr. Shetty was not an embryologist as he claimed to be and did not have the medical qualifications to run his sperm and egg banks, and surrogacy agency. Infertility doctors in the city with whom I'd conversed had also disparagingly said that Mr. Shetty was merely a "ward boy," someone who cleaned medical facilities, and did various small tasks under the employment of an established Bangalore infertility doctor. But Mr. Shetty maintained that he worked as an embryologist in this particular doctor's employment. Yet when asked, he was unable to say when and where he got his degree. He explained he had left this doctor's employment and begun the Creative Trust Options for Women in 2007 because he had established a reputation as someone who could recruit women for Bangalore's nascent reproductive assembly lines. By 2011 he ran three surrogacy dormitories each housing between ten and twelve women. He owned all these properties. He had done quite well for himself, considering his considerably short tenure in an industry fueled by working-class women's bodies.

The BBMP maintained that Mr. Shetty ran a trafficking business wherein surrogate mothers from among Bangalore's poor were enlisted to service wealthy clientele. On May 27, 2011, the Bangalore High Court directed COTW not to recruit any more surrogate mothers until investigations of COTW's licensing procedures were complete and COTW was legally cleared. However, the stream of egg donors and surrogate mothers continued to flow in and out of COTW's premises; I met women that summer who had been freshly recruited in spite of the legally mandated moratorium. The law was a mere suggestion and the only difference now was that Mr. Shetty was more careful about how he went about recruitment. Nothing seemed to stop his lucrative business.

If Mr. Shetty went around the law, I went around the moratorium he set on my research. I continued to interview egg donors and surrogate mothers; often these women had donated eggs just the previous week. Or the mothers were still residents in the dormitory, but were able to sneak out to meet with me at surrogate mother Salma's home where we'd eat mangoes, have lunch, drink sweet tea, and chat all day. All of us were engaging in subterfuge. His business dealings were furtive and illegal. The mothers broke COTW rules by meeting with me. And my research operations were clandestine as far as Mr. Shetty was concerned.

By 2012 Creative Options Trust for Women changed its name to Creative Global Medicare and Research Foundation. Along with supporting medical specialists in Bangalore, Mysore, and Chennai who provide infertility assistance, COTW's website claims that it continues its "charitable" work as before. In its latest iteration COTW supposedly provides shelter to newborn orphans from all over India, adoption assistance to childless couples, protection of girl babies, training for women toward self-employment, places women in employment, provides working women hostel services, gives widows and women divorcees employment and marriage assistance, provides free AIDS counseling and treatment, assists physically challenged individuals, and organizes blood donation camps, free eye clinics, and dental hygiene camps.

Sarita's first story—of the jealous girlfriend ousting her from COTW—was entirely credible. Yet now Sarita was telling me a considerably different story. Perhaps she had been embarrassed to reveal her employer's depravity and thought I'd judge her because she continued to work there in spite of sexual harassment? She was so distraught by this story she told me that it seemed truer than the first version. I felt terrible for having precipitated her calamities.

I called Sarita the following morning to find out how she was. She had not succeeded in making arrangements to repay Mr. Shetty because her alleged boyfriend was out of town. She began crying uncontrollably, saying that Mr. Shetty was going to return at 5:00 p.m. Could I give her $200 to bail her out? The $300 I had given her earlier in the week had gone to pay her mother's hospital bills, she said. She pleaded that I not tell anyone, especially my father, because she was ashamed of her troubles.

I returned home to Texas by the end of March 2011 feeling overwhelmed. Although I had managed to talk with some surrogate mothers, it seemed like my nascent research had been summarily halted because Mr. Shetty did not want me around any more. And on top of that I felt manipulated by Sarita. She unnerved me by heaping praise on me for which I had no reply: "For someone who comes from money you have no airs." And then she'd almost immediately jump to a putdown: "You people from America all wear such thick-strapped ugly sandals; why is that?" And she might add for good measure: "If you colored your hair you might actually appear attractive. Tell me truly, how old are you?" She told me contradictory stories. She narrated wild tales to others in my presence, but knew she could turn around and without batting an eyelid, request money from me. She had done a quick read and honed my liberal guilt to a fine degree, especially by constantly comparing my privileged upbringing to her difficult childhood. After forking over $1,000 to her in less than two weeks, I felt hustled.

She operated in ways that were antithetical to Bangalore's socially endorsed middle class mores; she exhibited a "mastery of a particular type of symbolic capital," such as the ability to get a quick read on her interlocutors, and deceive, manipulate, cajole, or charm them in order to achieve economic advantage.[3] If all else failed she threatened them and their loved ones with violence either inflicted by her or by others she knew because of her social and sexual intimacy with COTW's proprietor, Mr. Shetty. But over time I grew to appreciate all that Sarita had done. Without her assistance I would not have met any of the surrogate mothers. Why should she provide access to her contacts to me out of kindness just because I was some left-leaning America-returned feminist sociologist who wanted to write about Bangalore's surrogate mothers and their gendered oppression? A true exchangist, she would do something for me if I did something for her. If I had imagined her as a hustler, then by the end of 2011 it was impossible not to recognize that I too had benefited from her knowledge and her networks. From being an ethnographer of reproductive hustling, I as ethnographer had become a hustler. I used my extended social networks to exercise a kind of research entrepreneurialism to get the stories I wanted. To pretend otherwise was to engage in self-deception.

Over the course of the year Sarita became enormously angry with me, Roopa, and Suma, who were key recruiters of surrogate mothers. She had introduced them to me but now I met them in her absence. Sarita wanted me to pay her each time she took me to meet Roopa and Suma. Moreover, she demanded a cut of the money I gave to Roopa and Suma as "finder's fees." Roopa and Suma were unwilling to part with their hard-earned money. Potentially reliable sources in her erratic cash flow had closed down and Sarita was clearly unhappy that I met with Roopa and Suma without her supervision. She called on them unexpectedly to check if I'd made a telephone call or visited them. But I had established my own working relationships and did not need her assistance. Perhaps Sarita had made a good wager by getting as much as she could out of me while she could.

Roopa lived four blocks down the street from Sarita and had become entangled in Sarita's world when her daughter began attending evening tutorials with Sarita's mother a few years earlier. The child now took dance classes with Sarita three times a week. In addition, Roopa herself was recruited into becoming a surrogate mother three years earlier because of Sarita. I became privy to the fraught relationship between the two women by accident. One evening, when Umesha was driving me toward Roopa's we saw Sarita outside in her yard. In a phone call earlier she'd said she would be in Ooty, a vacation destination in the neighboring state of Tamil Nadu. She was apparently there on work as an external examiner to proctor an exam in her capacity as lecturer in a college in Bangalore. She was startled to see me when we stopped to exchange pleasantries. Why didn't you call me you were coming? she asked. I apologized, saying I was on my way to meet Roopa, and inquired about her recent trip. Sarita was visibly shaken. She quickly hushed me and said I was not to say another word about Ooty; her family did not know she had gone there. After chatting some more I told her I was running late, and giving her hands a tight squeeze, I left.

In the five minutes it took me to get to Roopa's house Sarita had already called, screaming at her, calling her a double-crosser and a whore. Roopa was in tears. She explained that Sarita and Mr. Shetty had a very close relationship. She was not proctoring an exam in Ooty; instead she was vacationing there with Mr. Shetty. She worried that Sarita would tell Mr. Shetty about our clandestine meetings and did not want to attract his wrath. Roopa also worried that Sarita would be verbally abusive toward her daughter during dance instruction. And finally, she worried that Sarita would cancel her orders of costumes she'd commissioned Roopa to sew for her dance school performances.

It was becoming apparent that Roopa, Sarita, and Mr. Shetty's worlds were deeply entangled. The surrogate mothers and egg donors, including Roopa and Sarita, loathed Mr. Shetty but needed him, held him in deference, yet expressed deep contempt in the very next breath. Suma had once said to me, "Mr. Shetty is like a god to us. If he were not here what would we do for money?" For the women he was not a benevolent god, but a malevolent one who brought fear, intimidation, and perhaps sexual coercion into their worlds. Along with that, he also brought the potential to make money.

If the women feared Mr. Shetty, then Roopa feared Sarita because of the latter's proximity to him. The two women's relationship exemplified recruiter-recruitee associations in Bangalore's reproductive industry. They were thickly bound together in a loose confederation of overlapping social groups. They were sisters, aunts, cousins twice removed, childhood friends, neighbors, coworkers, or their mothers had worked in the garment industry together; the links were endless. They kept tabs on each other, judged each others' actions, and attempted to create sanctions by cutting off economic opportunities, verbal abuse, and threats of physical violence through their ties to Mr. Shetty. Bangalore's reproductive market worked effectively because of these noneconomic associations laced with fear, shame, loyalty, honor, friendship, and love, which sometimes seemed to exist all at once.

The reproductive labor market was governed by nonmarket relations; if and when women broke their contracts they faced social consequences. So they adhered to industrial labor practices, especially sticking to the discipline imposed by labor contracts. Far from being an abstract, rational, unemotional, and open system that succeeded because of legal regulations and predictability that governed exchange, the reproductive assembly line worked effectively because of extralegal coercion, social pressures, and mutual reciprocal, hierarchical relationships instituted *a priori*, before the agents encountered each other in the marketplace. These were established, long-term ongoing social relationships, and the reproductive market simply became one more platform on which the women interacted in both economic and social ways.

Roopa: Recruitment through Friendship and Caring

Roopa, a single mother in her early thirties, was strikingly attractive but she did not believe herself to be so because her body was ravaged by vitiligo, an autoimmune disease that had left small, prominent white patches near her lips, eyes, and arms. Her family were of the land owning, dominant Gowda caste which did not necessarily translate to Roopa's family's economic status. Roopa's father had died at a young age, and her mother, a flower seller in the city market, raised three daughters and two sons on her own. Roopa was the youngest child in the family and had received a high school diploma before her marriage was arranged to a man who turned out to be a terrible husband and even worse father to their now nine-year-old daughter. Though her husband had left her, she was not alone; her natal family cared for her in a multitude of ways, right from buying her daughter little gifts to visiting her often.

Roopa had never sold her eggs, but was a surrogate mother in 2008, for which she had earned a mere $2,000. "I had no common sense," she said laughing, "I gave away all that money to my good-for-nothing, scheming husband." Yet she spent countless afternoons telling me she wanted to get back together with her estranged husband. "He's a very nice looking man, *akka*," she'd say. And he was a good man too; but he came from the neighboring Kollegal district where people practiced black magic. Roopa believed her husband had been bewitched, so she frequented neighborhood temples, visited local holy men, and made all sorts of religious vows to dispel the sinister spells cast on her husband. She wanted him back because she said it was very hard to live as a respectable thirty-five-year-old woman without a husband. She also worried for her daughter. Would her future marriage alliances be affected if families got to know that her mother was separated and possibly divorced? For much of our time together, Roopa schemed in this world and crusaded against spirits of the netherworld to have her spouse returned to her.[4]

During the countless times I visited, Roopa would insist that Umesha, the young man who chauffeured me in Bangalore, park the car as far away as possible from her home so Sarita and Mr. Shetty's men would not know I was visiting. For additional security we'd walk away from her home through labyrinthine alleys to reach her garment worker friend Madhavi's house where I'd meet with interviewees she'd recruited. At these times Umesha would worry for my safety. "You must carry your phone with you at all times, *akka*," he'd say, taking my cell phone from my hands and turning up the ringer volume to the highest level before returning it to me. These working-class neighborhoods felt unpredictable and unsafe, where life had a discounted market value, where human kidneys and eggs, wombs, and babies were trafficked on a daily basis. I had located myself smack in the middle of this human trafficking, engaging in my own petty trade in information. But with Roopa I felt safe.

We'd sit barefoot and cross-legged on her spotless living room floor in her three-room home. This front room, which doubled as her work space, was dominated by a large, sparkling clean fish tank, a television, and a sewing machine. Half-sewn and completed garments were separated into neatly folded piles on the floor and the two plastic chairs by the front door. Over glasses of overly sweetened coffee, store-bought cookies, and occasional home-cooked spicy mutton curries that brought tears of pain to my eyes—much to Roopa's endless mirth—we'd share stories of making ends meet, what we wanted for our daughters' futures, and for ourselves. Or we'd argue over politics. Roopa was a voracious reader, devouring Kannada print media and occasionally English news magazines.

Roopa's home was always busy. Someone would stop by either to chat or request a custom-made sari blouse. Neighborhood children often came in the evenings to eat cookies, drink a glass of milk, and attend to homework under Roopa's supervision before their mothers returned home from work in garment factories. A six-year-old boy, who was always at her home, was her closest friend, garment worker Madhavi's only child. He considered Roopa his second mother. Madhavi's husband was having an extramarital affair and she often asked Roopa to intervene because he listened only to her. Roopa would lovingly reprimand Madhavi that a man who could not keep his promises was useless. She had to leave him. And then she'd look over at me and mirthfully say that the two women spent so much time together that neighbors joked that they were married; Roopa was the husband and Madhavi, the wife.

As with most of the women I met, Roopa's monthly income was elastic. She preferred not to work in garment factories anymore. The supervisor in the last factory she had worked at had touched her inappropriately and she lost her temper. She soundly reprimanded him and quit work that very day. "The men there do not have good character," she said as her face contorted with contempt. In her experience as a garment worker, sexual degradation was the principal way by which women were compelled to work almost without a break on the shop floor in order to extract maximum labor effort. The only way to stop sexual harassment in garment factories, she often said, was to replace all male supervisors with women. Since that was not possible, she did piecework at home for small factories. This way she worked at her own pace and was there for her daughter when she came back from school. This was important for Roopa because the child was nine years old, and from Roopa's perspective ripe for sexual abuse by neighbors and acquaintances.

Roopa also taught tailoring classes to women in the neighborhood who wanted to pursue work in garment factories. In addition, she sewed made-to-order sari blouses for women and dresses for girls in the neighborhood.[5] With vitiligo patches on her face, which developed *after* she had been a surrogate mother three years earlier, Roopa was now ineligible for surrogacy and egg donation. Instead she recruited egg donors and surrogate mothers for COTW. It was easy to see why Roopa was an effective recruiter; not only had she been a surrogate mother before and could personally attest to what that entailed, but in addition she had charisma. She was fierce, and she was confident. As she walked purposefully down the street she called out happy greetings to people and inquired after their workday or health. Though separated from her husband and living as a single woman with her nine-year-old daughter, she was considered very proper and was held in high regard by the people who lived around her. As a result, they conducted themselves decorously in her presence.

The other recruiters I'd met extracted a small payment from interviewees for having been introduced to me, but Roopa refused to take money from them unless they offered her a gift. This "lost opportunity," however, was not in vain. What she lost in finances she more than made up in building trust networks. These interviews I conducted were just another way by which Roopa provided opportunities for women in her neighborhood to make money. It was actions such as these that made Roopa an honorable person in their eyes. Women came to her with their troubles and she sought to assist them either by advising their families to treat them better, or connecting them to others she knew who might assist them. It was not surprising that she was the top recruiter of egg donors and surrogate mothers for COTW, drawing mainly from garment workers, construction workers, and a few *agarbathi* (incense sticks) workers.

I met most of the egg donors through Roopa.[6] She also recruited a large number of surrogate mothers to be interviewed by me.[7] Through conversations with women in Roopa's and Madhavi's homes I learned so much about how women got embroiled in markets in life. I reproduce here one such story that is especially illustrative of how women found themselves on Bangalore's reproductive assembly lines.

The Social Value of Women

An oft-repeated refrain in my conversations with the surrogate mothers was, "*Dhudu idha rene namage bele.*" That is, they declared they have social value only if they possessed money.[8] I met with Vijaya and Nagu in Roopa's house one Sunday morning when the women were not at work in the garment factories. The three women were neighbors and Roopa had recruited them to be surrogate mothers over a year earlier. Vijaya and Nagu were roommates in the COTW dormitory, and, like Roopa, belonged to the Gowda caste. When they saw me at Roopa's and were not at work, they'd come over and the four of us would have long conversations. In that first conversation, which is one of the few I recorded, Vijaya began speaking in Kannada: "I have had a difficult life. I am from Shimoga. My father died when my younger brother was still in my mother's womb. So she brought me to Bangalore to be employed as a child care worker for a respectable family. I was just ten years old when I was separated from my mother. She could not feed me."

Because her mother could barely make ends meet as a landless agricultural laborer, and because she was fatherless and therefore unprotected and vulnerable to sexual abuse, Vijaya was married off at sixteen to a relative who lived in Bangalore. Two years later she gave birth to a daughter, and at twenty-one she had her son, after which she opted to get permanently sterilized. "I wanted more children," she said, but her husband thought that two children were enough because of their economic circumstances. Vijaya said, "I struggle for them. All that I do is for my children. And I send money to Shimoga. Poor thing, my mother is not getting any younger. I also want my brother educated. He is only fifteen years old."

Realizing we were soon talking about finding funding for her brother's education and not surrogacy, I interjected, "So you were a surrogate mother . . . when?" Vijaya replied, "One year ago. Roopa saw my struggles and took me to COTW." She had taken on a loan of $2,000 to make a security deposit on the house they were renting. She also needed money to enroll her children in private school. And finally, she wanted a good education for her younger brother who wanted to teach in a small-town college. She added, "My husband didn't take responsibility for the loan. He is an alcoholic. He drinks too much. He beats me too. Look at me," she said, gesturing at the third-degree burns on her forearms. They had gotten into a fight. He'd picked up burning wood from the stove to beat her, but she had managed to stop him. He had gotten burned too. "He burned me all over my arm three days ago. But I can't leave him because the children need him. He is a good father. I need that money he makes to help with the children. But I need more so I'll sell my eggs for $500." At this point Roopa cut in:

> *Akka*, a man is not like us women. He has *bele* [social worth or value]. He goes out of the house and earns money . . . even if he is out of the house at all odds hours of the night, no one says anything. . . . In fact, his social value grows because people will say that he has even sacrificed his sleep in order to earn money for his family. But if a woman does this the very same people cast aspersions. What is she doing out of the house at night, they will ask. Is she a prostitute? There is only so much we as women can do to earn money.

Vijaya added that it was difficult to engage in wage employment outside the home. People slandered her, questioning her character and her sexual morals because she was away from the chaperoning protection of family and interacting in public spaces with men who were not kinfolk. On the other hand, it was hard to stay home without wages too. Their husbands often accused them of being lazy because they ostensibly did nothing at home but cook, eat, and otherwise have a leisurely life. Their husbands did not recognize housework as legitimate work. "It hurts so much, but what answer can you give to that," Vijaya said. To which Nagu quickly replied, "No man can earn $4,000 in nine months and give it to his wife's hands. He can't." Commercialized pregnancy afforded her greater earnings because of her sex, which was unprecedented in her social world. Employment on Bangalore's reproduction industry put money in her hands and that, she felt, empowered her. It gave her *bele*.

The conversation drifted away, yet again, from how the women felt about surrogacy to Vijaya's everyday struggles. It was a pattern I would grow to recognize by the time I had talked with seventy women. They did not oblige me by talking only about surrogacy. I was never sure whether they avoided talking about surrogacy because their everyday lives were so fraught that their employment as surrogate mothers seemed distant and far away. Or did they feel no pain of separation from those surrogated babies, which then meant they'd be demonized for being unnatural women, and therefore they did not want to talk about their feelings? Or was the pain of having given up a baby they birthed so great that they kept quiet—to invoke that reality would open up the wounds all over again, making the loss seem so much harder because they could never put it to rest? I was never able to tell why they spoke reluctantly about surrogacy. So I'd interpose: "Tell me what you think about surrogacy. Was it a good or bad experience for you? How did you feel?"

Vijaya answered that she was of two minds. On one level she was glad because so much depended on the money she earned as a surrogate mother. Though she did not get to see the baby, hold her, or even know who took her, Vijaya was glad that the surrogated baby "will grow up with someone who has money. She will not face difficulties like my children do. I know those people who took her will take care of her, but inside me, I will always feel pain. I may feel relief about my money situation, but the pain is in my mind constantly." Nagu intervened: "The money disappears, *akka*. It is gone in months. But that pain? I live with it every single day." Nagu wondered whether the baby now had long hair. How tall might she be? Who did she look like? What made her smile? How often did she smile?

Roopa grieved about her separation from her surrogated baby. Unlike other surrogate mothers who delivered through caesarian sections, she had delivered vaginally. But she was not allowed to see or hold the baby girl who was taken away from almost the moment she was born. Roopa did not know who took the baby, or the little girl's current location. She said this secrecy was for her own good because it protected her from the pain that came from loving the little child, but also simultaneously knowing that baby could never be a part of her life. Yet she also believed that the child and she were a part of each other, and because of that the two of them were spiritually connected. Roopa commemorated the baby's birthday every year with delicacies she cooked at home. She believed that because the baby had grown in her womb, she would have imbibed Roopa's character and life values. She mourned that she would never have another child and felt guilty that she had deprived her own daughter of a baby sister. Roopa said, "The egg is not mine. That is true. But I have borne that baby in my womb for nine months. If something were to happen to my daughter, then that child I have given up is the only child I have left. I want her in my life."

Nagu interrupted, "When your troubles are over, you forget the money you have earned. That money is gone forever from your hands. All that remains is the memory of that baby. And when you have pain like that you know you will repay the money. Really, if I could I would give them their money back. Somehow. Perhaps take a loan. But I want my baby back."

Nagu, Vijaya, and Roopa all said that the loss they felt was not just for themselves, but also for their children. Vijaya articulated that she felt especially sad when she saw her children play with each other. "Would this baby have played with them too? And how would she play with her older sister and brother? How would my children be different because of this little baby in their lives?" Surrogacy was a loss for some mothers, for their children, and the surrogated child who had "lost" siblings. Many women felt guilty they had deprived *all* the children they had birthed.

"But who do you talk with, *akka*," said Nagu. "We can't express ourselves to anyone. First of all, my neighbors don't know I've been a surrogate mother. My parents and siblings don't either. And even if they did, they would not understand this pain. How can they know what it was like to give birth to a baby and then give her up? The pain is constant in my mind, but I must continue to live every day."

Such was the tenor of conversations I had with women I met through Roopa. Roopa had strong bonds of friendship with them. She identified with their pains and struggles. She tended their emotional and physical wounds. She fought for them with their husbands, in-laws, and employers if she felt they had been wronged. She worked on a keen sense of right and wrong, voicing vociferously the injustices at work and at home. And because of that, a vast group of women trusted her. If she said employment at COTW was a worthwhile endeavor, they believed her. If she empathized with them, saying that giving up the surrogated baby was devastating but they had to earn money in order to have *bele*, the women believed her. After all, that was Roopa's lived experience and she exemplified what she preached. She had an unwavering moral ethos by which she conducted her own life and the women strongly identified with that.

Markets *and* Intimacy

Sociologist Viviana Zelizer observes that markets and intimacy are deeply imbricated in each other because "economic activity is an integral and essential part of a wide range of intimate relations [and] the presence of intimacy endows the economic activity with special significance."[9] People manage the intrusion of social life into markets by performing "relational work."[10] Thus they distinguish between different kinds of child care, for example, such as mother care, grandparent babysitting, and professional child care, each of which comes with its own set of rights, obligations, and compensatory systems. Zelizer admonishes us that "we should stop agonizing over whether or not money corrupts, but instead analyze what combinations of economic activity and intimate relations produce happier, more just, and more productive lives. It is not the mingling that should concern us, but how the mingling works."[11]

Taking her seriously, I show that labor markets in surrogate mothers in Bangalore emerge from networks of women residing in garment district neighborhoods. Social intimacy and labor markets were thickly intertwined. Established personal interconnections among women enabled them to coax and convince each other that vending their eggs and marketing their pregnancy were worthwhile economic endeavors. Emergent marketable reproductive labor was embedded in social principles that were commonly shared and already in circulation. Women's worth was already established. Compensatory systems, *bakshish*, and gift giving already existed, and it was within these rules and regulations that Mr. Shetty, Roopa, Sarita, and other recruiters operated. This commingling of social intimacy and markets did not necessarily produce more happiness or more justice, but it certainly made available a large pool of workers who complied with the bodily discipline so central to the efficiency of Bangalore's reproductive assembly lines.

Recruiting for Markets in Life

Scholars note that labor markets are not abstract social systems but are rooted in local cultural practices and contain unspoken expectations based on trust, in which moral economies outside the workplace form the basis of interactions at work.[12] The labor market for surrogate mothers was much like that; it did not exist *a priori* but was socially emergent.

Just because new forms of employment, in this case egg "donation" and surrogacy, existed did not mean that women wanted to pursue such work. They needed to feel *inclined* to engage in this opportunity to make money. But in order to feel that inclination two developments had to occur; first, potential workers needed to learn about egg "donation" and surrogacy, and second, they needed to trust their employer.

COTW was very efficient at educating Bangaloreans about egg donation and surrogacy; Mr. Shetty advertised his employment services over Kannada television, radio, and Kannada newspapers.[13] Yet women may have wondered, What kind of work was this? Who were the employers? Were they trustworthy? It was here that recruiting agents entered the scene. They mediated between potential workers and employers by screening suitable employees and bringing them to the shop floor. And they taught workers to develop the discipline required on reproductive assembly lines.

To describe how these markets in life work, I borrow two terms from postindustrial production to explain the crucial roles recruiting agents played; these are just-in-time production and pyramid schemes. Just-in-time (JIT) production is key to postindustrial production regimes where unused inventory is minimized to save costs. Taiichi Ohno and his Toyota Motor Company colleagues pioneered the process in the post–World War II era. To work around the logistics associated with storing and then moving inventory, "Ohno and his colleagues introduced a system in which no part . . . was made until the ultimate customer or the next stage in the production process specifically requested it."[14] Storage of unused raw materials and parts already produced consumed resources that could be used elsewhere. Clients' requirements too could change and thus inventory could be wasted. Calling it the "complete elimination of waste," Toyota describes JIT in the following manner:

> "Just-in-Time" means making "only what is needed, when it is needed, and in the amount needed." For example, to efficiently produce a large number of automobiles, which can consist of around 30,000 parts, it is

> necessary to create a detailed production plan that includes parts procurement. Supplying "what is needed, when it is needed, and in the amount needed" according to this production plan can eliminate waste, inconsistencies, and unreasonable requirements, resulting in improved productivity.[15]

Because the reproduction industry deals with human eggs and surrogate mothers, storage is not feasible. Many clients need to select egg donors. And they need to select surrogate mothers. Producing a surrogacy pregnancy and eventually a baby requires a tremendous amount of coordination. Two women's bodies need to be stimulated with synthetic hormones; egg extraction is coordinated with preparing the surrogate mother's body just in time to facilitate a successful assisted conception.

Given its trade in human bodies and living tissues, COTW is unable to ascertain its assets in raw materials or the amount of stock it sits on because such inventory cannot be held. However, when needed the right bodily material must be summoned at the right time and in the right amounts, to the right place. In order to achieve such coordination, COTW maintained rosters of women who were ready to make their bodies available for egg harvesting or surrogacy as and when needed. The most effective way for COTW to maintain networks of women who could be quickly incorporated into reproductive assembly lines was through recruitment agents. COTW was a model neoliberal firm; with very few actual employees on its payroll it was able to muster a sizable workforce of women in prime reproductive age when needed. And when the work was done, the women, who were treated like "independent contractors," were moved out of the firm's premises and payroll. Under these circumstances the firm bore very few overhead costs for the maintenance of the workforce, while simultaneously reducing the risks to itself. The risks were all borne by individual women, those "independent contractors" who vended their services when and where needed.

All the recruiting agents were former egg donors and surrogate mothers themselves. Successful recruiters tended to be women who were prominent in their neighborhoods and who had worked to build networks with a wide range of women from whom they recruited. Women on Bangalore's reproductive assembly lines signed on not because they trusted Mr. Shetty; instead, they had established ongoing social engagements with recruiting agents and were drawn in by thick and thin multiple bonds based on familiarity, fear, and trust. The recruitment of egg donors and surrogate mothers in Bangalore was organized much like a pyramid scheme. Otherwise called a form of "multi-level marketing," pyramid schemes worked by converting social networks into marketing networks.[16] Those selling Amway products, for example, receive a commission "not just for each unit sold, but also for the 'downline'—the new tiers of sellers whom the sales force recruits and from whom they also receive a commission for every unit sold."[17] Recruitment worked in much the same way. Take the case of Sarita: because she had recruited Roopa, she earned a nominal sum of money on each of Roopa's recruitees. Thus, each recruiting agent continued to earn money (at whatever nominal rate, like most pyramid schemes) because some of their recruitees in turn recruited others into reproductive assembly lines. All they needed to do was keep tabs on each other and protect their "turf" so that other recruiters would not encroach on their networks.

The women believed the reproductive industry could deliver them from economic precarity. They said so repeatedly. Yet the women never made enough money to move out of their economic desperation. On the other hand, Mr. Shetty, as originator of this pyramid scheme of recruitment, had accumulated vast capital in Bangalore through his proprietary claims on reproductive assembly lines. Thus, recruitment in surrogacy worked like a pyramid scheme in more ways than one—not only did it rely on converting social networks into market networks, but the women never earned enough to be economically self-sufficient. On the other hand, the originator of the scheme, Mr. Shetty, amassed considerable wealth.

3

The Many Meanings of Surrogacy

Suma: The Relentless Struggle to Enjoy the Good Life

When we first met, Suma was six months pregnant and living in the surrogacy dormitory. Unlike others, who were crowded into one small room for four, Suma had only one other roommate whom I never met because she had just delivered her baby and left. Suma had a big personality; if the corridors between the rooms were dirty, she would object loudly, take a broom, and commence to clean the floors. COTW staff could not slack off when Suma was around. Her fellow residents at the dormitory appreciated her ability to protest and make demands. Prabha, Indirani's sister who had stayed on as a surrogate mother long after Suma left the dorm, complained, "The food, Suma! I can't put it in my mouth. It's not like when you had taken over the kitchen."

For much of her stay at the surrogacy dormitory Suma had appointed herself head chef at the kitchen facilities. The staff had been relegated to line cook status, and different mothers were assigned to chop vegetables or clean out the rice as the need arose. I ate lunch every day with the residents when I was allowed on the premises. Suma would beam from ear to ear as she heaped food on my plate, saying, "I'm so glad you got to eat food made with my hands. I'm a good cook. Aren't I? Here, eat some more." This was no idle boasting. She was. Suma asserted that good food was essential to a good life. "I may be poor, *akka*," she'd say, "but I will not eat like a poor person. Why struggle so much if we can't enjoy life?"

Suma told me she was thirty years old, married, and worked from home. Unlike other interviews, where I interjected regularly to get details about dates and such, Suma spoke at length with hardly any interruptions. Suma had two sisters, and because their alcoholic father had abandoned the family, the mother returned to her maternal home and raised them with the help of her extended family. Their family had migrated from Tamil Nadu to Bangalore a few generations ago, and though they were Gownders by caste, they hardly spoke any Tamil. By Bangalore's standards the family was comfortable because they owned their home. Suma's mother and her aunts had been garment workers almost from the time the factories first started popping up in the city. Suma's school was close to the factory; after school, she'd meet her mother up at the factory and they'd walk home together. Suma's mother was very eager to have her educated, so she got her admission at a local college to major in science because she wanted her daughter to be a doctor. But Suma met her future husband, who insisted he could not wait; so she quit her studies and married him at nineteen. They were both Tamilian and of the Gownder caste, but because they had married without parental blessings they had to start a new household, which was very expensive. They had never fully recovered from the financial burdens of their early days of marriage, yet Suma was very happy with her choices because she said she was blessed with three sons. The oldest one was eight years old and the youngest was three. Her youngest sister, who did not have any children of her own, was raising Suma's middle child, who was five.

Because Suma was at the dormitory, her friend Mangala was taking care of her two sons and receiving $20 monthly for her troubles.[1] Suma felt that being a surrogate mother would help her be a better mother to her sons. She needed the money because she and her husband had taken a loan to buy an auto rickshaw. However, their vehicle was repossessed because their friend, who had borrowed it, did not make the down payments on the auto rickshaw. Suma had also pawned all the jewelry she had received from her mother. She was determined to get her jewelry back and buy another auto rickshaw. She said:

> I don't care if I drink *ganji* [rice porridge made with water and salt] every day, but I don't want these loans on my head. I don't want a lot of money. What to do with that much money? I'm not going to take it with me when

> I die. I want two things—I want to enjoy life and I want to fulfill my duties toward my children. My mother single-handedly got three children educated in an English-medium school. Before my mother died in 2007 she told me: Look, without a husband I have got you educated in an English-medium school. You have not lacked anything in life. Your good fortune is that you have borne only male children. I am not going to give you endless advice . . . but all I can say is this. You have to educate them well.

Unlike other surrogate mothers who made $4,000, the commissioning parents had slipped an additional $2,000 amidst the folds of the sari they'd gifted Suma. In addition they had given her a gold necklace as a "thank you" gift. Suma believed she received these gifts because she had birthed a baby boy for them. If Mr. Shetty and his staff got to know of these gifts, Suma said, they would have kept them for themselves and she would not have received a penny.

In spite of her earnings and the commission she made from recruitment, Suma's financial woes were endless. She paid off her loans of $2,000 and retrieved her jewelry from the pawnshop. She bought a new television and a TV stand to house it on. She also gifted her husband a brand new motorbike, which was subsequently stolen. The last time we met Suma was going to various police stations to recover the stolen bike. And she was receiving hormonal shots to become a surrogate mother all over again so she could build a savings account. She truly believed that surrogacy could pull her out of her precarious financial situation. She often said that Mr. Shetty was like "a god" to her and her family. He provided when all else failed.

Salma: Converting Money into Social Power

Salma was three months pregnant when we met in March 2011.[2] I became reacquainted with her through Suma, and met her frequently when she was much further along in her pregnancy. Her home was close to the dormitory and she received permission to return home often. I interviewed other COTW residents who'd accompany her on her forays back home. Salma was the twenty-two-year-old daughter of a garment worker, with a two-year-old son of her own. A practicing Sayyid Muslim woman, she married a Hindu man she met at the garment factory. Until the birth of her son both her in-laws and her parents disapproved of her marriage. Now, however, her in-laws raised her son in their village home 150 kilometers away while she and her husband worked in the garment factory.

Salma's husband was unhappy that she was a surrogate mother and wanted to go back to the village to live with his parents. They could help his parents in their agricultural work, and he and Salma could save money because they would not have to maintain a home in Bangalore. But Salma wanted to live in the city where she had grown up, far from the eyes of prying relatives.

As the Muslim wife of the middle son in a Hindu family, she had come into the marital household with no bargaining power. She did not have parental support in her marital choice either, which further weakened her social status. Surrogacy, she felt, facilitated her negotiations within her extended family. A large proportion of the $4,000 she earned through surrogacy would go toward assisting her Hindu in-laws. To increase crop yields they had got two bore wells drilled, and Salma and her husband had borne that expenditure through borrowed money. Her earnings through surrogacy would repay that loan. By investing her earnings back into ancestral property, small as the holdings were, she had solidified her standing in her marital Hindu family, significantly establishing herself as a contributing and therefore worthy member in spite of being a practicing Muslim woman. Salma's possession of money established her social worth or her *bele*.

Indirani: Loving Children Is Hard Work for the Poor

Married at eighteen, and with two young children of her own, Indirani had delivered twins in June 2011 for a Tamil couple in the United States.[3] I first met Indirani and her older sister, Prabha, in the dormitory during my first visit to Bangalore. I was later reintroduced to her through Suma, with whom she had a conflicted relationship because their networks overlapped and they recruited from more or less the same "pools" of women; like Suma, the sisters were Gownder. Indirani had recruited her two sisters into surrogacy. The younger sister, Kavita, was a single mother of three children. She had attempted surrogacy three times previously but had miscarried each time. She had already begun recruiting women even before becoming a surrogate mother herself. Their mother helped the two sisters with their brokerage services. It had become a family business. Kavita was determined to become a surrogate mother; she was pregnant the fourth time around and in COTW in December 2011.

Indirani's "regular" job was at the garment factory. Just as Roopa had done earlier, she too spoke of male supervisors on the garment shop floor who castigated women in sexually derogatory terms when they did not meet production quotas. Indirani said she would not take lunch breaks when garment pieces piled up because she did not want to draw the supervisors' unwanted attention. Frequently she and her coworkers had to stay past regular working hours to meet the inordinately high production targets. "Playing" catch-up, however, did not result in overtime pay. During these times Indirani's husband suspected her of marital fidelity; if she was working overtime, as she claimed she was, then why wasn't she getting paid overtime? She earned $100 to $110 monthly, depending on attendance and punctuality, and in rare instances, overtime pay.

Indirani and her auto rickshaw driver husband struggled to make ends meet. He rented his vehicle from an acquaintance, and the daily rental and gasoline costs cut significantly into their income. So Indirani and he decided to borrow money from her cousin to purchase an auto rickshaw of their own, but they were unable to pay off the loan. Her cousin, the moneylender, would verbally abuse them and come by the garment factory on payday each month and take Indirani's entire paycheck. She said, "I'd work hard, facing all sorts of abuse. And at the end of it I wouldn't even see any money. I felt so bad I contemplated suicide." When a friend at work suggested that she sell her eggs for approximately

$500, Indirani felt hope. After "donating" her eggs, Indirani decided to try surrogacy, and was pregnant with twins at the very first attempt.

Soon after, Mr. Shetty called her into his office and said, "Look *amma*, you may be pregnant with twins and think you deserve more. But do not desire money. Take what the parents give you and be content with that. Wanting more, asking for more will only leave you feeling bitter and everyone unhappy." Even if she was legally entitled to a larger amount because she birthed twins, Indirani made no more than those mothers pregnant with singletons. Her commissioning parents had given her a substantially bigger amount as a "thank you" gift, but she never received a single penny of it. Her take-home pay was less than $4,000 after she paid the recruiting agent $200 and bought small, obligatory gifts for the COTW staff because they had taken care of her during her pregnancy. Indirani had the option of staying on in the dormitory for up to two months after delivering her twins through caesarian section, but like all the mothers I met, she chose not to because COTW would charge her for postnatal care, food, and board. So she returned home, and within a week her remaining earnings went to the moneylender. She had no money left, but knowing her debts were paid off gave her peace of mind. Yet she needed to build her savings. She said:

> If you asked me two years ago whether I'd have a baby and give it away for money, I wouldn't just laugh at you, I would be so insulted I might hit you in the face. Yet here I am today. I carried those twin babies for nine months and gave them up. Do you know anyone who wants a surrogate mother? I need to do this again.

Kavita, Indirani's youngest sister and a single mother, who was not yet successfully pregnant in spite of three surrogacy attempts, said she loved babies. "I am crazy about them, madam. I have three of my own and if I could have more I would! But my husband and I are not together any more. I think I will run after those parents, hold their feet, and beg them to let me hold the baby. I don't know how I will find the strength [to give up the baby] when my time comes." Indirani was annoyed by her youngest sister's mawkishness. She exasperatedly said that women needed to think about their own dependent children. If there was no market for reproduction how would they earn money to support their families? She turned to me and said, "To be truthful, madam. I do not have even a sesame seed of desire for those twin babies."[4] She advised her coresidents in the dormitory to not desire the baby they carried.

While it may very well have been the case that Indirani had no affection for the babies she birthed, I was struck by the frequency with which she repeated two Kannada phrases that loosely translate as the following: "Do not desire the baby," and she did not have "a sesame seed" of love for the babies she had carried. She repeated these exact phrases so often that I came to realize that Indirani *worked* hard to be unsentimental and distanced herself from the twins she had birthed. In one of our numerous meetings, she said to me, "For the poor like us it is difficult to love children. When you love children you must work so hard for them. Why do you think I am doing all this right now? It is to raise my children. . . . So that my daughter will never have to make the kinds of choices I have made. I want more for her life than I have had. I work hard now and pray that she will never become a surrogate mother."

Prabha: The Sentimental Sister

If Indirani wanted to appear hard-nosed and calculating, her older sister Prabha and younger sister Kavita were just the opposite. They wore their hearts on their sleeves. Thirty-two-year-old Prabha's friends at COTW, that is, her sister and Suma, had already given birth to babies and left. She felt alone and bored because she had not developed strong bonds with the current dormitory residents. She couldn't wait to give birth to her surrogated baby and return to her home in Kolar, which was about 70 kilometers outside Bangalore. Prabha said nothing about her pregnancy and the fetus she bore within her. Instead, her immense sentimentality was directed toward her in-laws.

Prabha's was an arranged marriage. At seventeen years of age her parents had gotten her married to her maternal cousin.[5] Because she and her husband lived in a joint family, where multiple generations live together in the same household, Prabha was embedded in her mother's natal family encompassed by her maternal uncle and maternal grandparents' fierce loving protection. Prabha's family doted on her and she in turn was devoted to their well-being. She had entered into surrogacy in order to help make improvements to their agricultural holdings. Her family was grateful to her for her efforts. They missed her, and she in turn longed for them, especially her aging maternal uncle/father-in-law. He was hospitalized because he had fallen and broken his leg. He needed surgery. She worried that being over seventy years old, he might not heal well. "He's in a lot of pain, madam," she said. "He is too old to suffer like this. Poor man. He asks for me. I want to go be with him." She longed to go back home to her extended family. She knew her children were loved and nurtured and did not worry about them; and she did not even talk of the fetus she carried within her because this child would leave her life. Instead, for the duration of the entire interview she spoke about how she missed the older folk in her family, and how she wanted to return to take care of them.

Chitra: Love Does Not Come Cheap

If Prabha was adored and doted on by her marital extended family, twenty-three-year-old Chitra had the opposite experience. She met the love of her life at work in the garment factory and married him, much to her mother-in-law's ire. Her mother-in-law alleged that her son had wasted his economic opportunities by marrying Chitra because he could have received a hefty dowry from someone else. As a result, she berated her son constantly and was contemptuous of Chitra. Even upon the birth of her son—a grandson for the older woman—Chitra felt her mother-in-law's derision. She felt her mother-in-law would never accept her until she got a large dowry.[6] So when Kavita offered her a chance, she gladly jumped into surrogacy. By earning $4,000 Chitra believed she could earn her mother-in-law's approval.

Receiving Wages for Pregnancy: What Does It Mean?

For much of her career Arlie Hochschild has focused on the deepening commodification of emotions.[7] Her recent book, *The Outsourced Self* (2012) examines the invasion of the market into intimate spheres of life—love coaches who guide internet dating, professional wedding planners, marriage therapists, outsourced pregnancy where the infertile use surrogacy services in India, nannies who raise children, and party planners for children's birthdays. She writes: "Even more than *what* we wish, the market alters *how* we wish. Wallet in hand, we focus in the market on the thing we want to buy. . . . What escapes us is the *process* of getting there—the appreciation we attach to the small details of it."[8] Hochschild believes that Americans have become a nation of outsourcers, which has resulted in degradation of community life.

Though Arlie Hochschild may not describe herself as doing so, in her current opus she continues to privilege the gift mode of exchange over commodity exchange, as in her earlier work. In her magisterial *The Managed Heart: The Commercialization of Feeling* she writes that private, nonmarket life is mediated by gifts of feeling, which are exchanged freely because individuals have independence and choice in questioning inequality in private life. If unhappy with "the going rate of exchange," they are "free to negotiate a new one." If not satisfied, they can leave, as witnessed by the "many friendships and marriages [that] die of inequality."[9] However, she despairs that "[w]e have carried our ancient capacity for gift exchange over a great commercial divide where gifts are becoming commodities and the exchange rates are set by corporations."[10] Because emotions now have exchange value, corporations control how workers emote. Workers are not free to reveal emotions that are authentic to their innermost selves; instead, they must follow company policies that regard the consumer as almost always right. As a result, care workers must accept unequal exchanges and "be treated with disrespect or anger by a client."[11] The gracious mutuality created by exchanging gifts comprised a mode of social integration that is rapidly being eroded under the onslaught of the market. Social isolation has led to marketization and perversely, increasing marketization has led to greater isolation. People attempt to keep the depersonalizing effects of the market at bay. Hochschild writes, "We avoid. We substitute. We compensate. We take back. We reach out. We subordinate. We can use several mechanisms of defense, serially or at the same time, or none at all."[12] But nothing halts the deepening marketization of private life. We attempt to control "the market from inside. [But] what we're not doing is altering the basic imbalance between market, state, and civic life that has caused us to draw line after line in the first place."[13]

Extending Hochschild's line of reasoning it is obvious that Bangalore's surrogate mothers turn to markets in life for emotional and physical sustenance because the other kind of employment available to them, namely, garment work, has become increasingly untenable. Their participation on reproductive assembly lines, however, leads to greater isolation. They are alienated from their labor, from the babies they birth, and from the consuming parents who take away newborn babies from them. Hochschild is absolutely correct at one level.

Yet she fails to recognize that gift giving is *not* a gender-neutral activity innocent of exploitation and dispossession. A different truth emerges when we replace the ostensibly egalitarian reciprocity of the gift exchange with the realities of women's unequal positions in societies and the debasement of their gendered activities. As anthropologist Marilyn Strathern explains, "[M]en's and women's ability to transact with this or that item stems from the power this gendering gives some persons at the expense of others, as does the necessity and burden of carrying through transactions."[14] Gift transactions mystify women's continuous input of labor in making socially useful things, which then get exchanged as gifts between men, families, and clans. Speaking of the Kewa in Melanesia, Strathern says, "a wife must feed all the pigs to which a husband lays claim, wherever they may come from, yet her labor does not necessarily establish any entitlement to them." The belief in the reciprocity of gift giving, Strathern says:

> perpetuates the myth that gifts create gifts. . . . It obscures inequalities in men's access to productive resources among themselves, since the ability to obtain gifts is seen not as a matter of number of wives or size of gardens but of skill in transactions. And in the case of pigs it obscures the considerable female labor that goes into their maintenance. Since only men gain a name, they convert material into symbolic capital while excluding women in the process.[15]

Women's labor that goes into the production of pigs, in this case, is appropriated in the interest of men. Those pigs belong to the husband who can sacrifice them in feasts. He is free to convert "his" material wealth into social capital. His wife too accrues social capital but only through her marital attachment to him. She is not able to negotiate in the political sphere and exchange these pigs that exist in large part because of her extensive effort. Women's labor in raising those pigs is acknowledged and even respected, but such effort does not belong solely to her. Her exertions are annexed to the patriarchal family, expropriated toward building power and status for the men who transact the pigs publicly.

Moreover, women themselves are exchanged as gifts, bequeathed from one family to another. As anthropologists note, "[O]ften gifts subsume persons themselves, especially under patrilineal regimes where women move in marriage from one set of men to another."[16] Feminist anthropologist Gayle Rubin astutely observes, "[T]he men who give and take them . . . are linked, the woman being a conduit of a relationship rather than a partner of it."[17] A father walks down the aisle to give away his daughter in marriage to another man. She loses her father's name and takes on her husband's. She is transferred from one family to another. The children she births bear their father's name. As Levi-Strauss so beautifully shows in *The Elementary Structures of Kinship*, the incest taboo, which varies so greatly from culture to culture, is not meant simply to perpetuate a human species with no "in breeding"; instead, the taboo insures that the exchange of women takes place between families, lineages, and clans. He writes: "The prohibition of incest is less a rule prohibiting marriage with the mother, sister, or daughter than a rule obliging the mother, sister or daughter to be given to others. It is the supreme rule of the gift."[18]

There is a long and sordid history in the "traffic in women." Women and their reproductive labors broadly defined—cooking, caring for families, birthing and raising children—have almost always been exchanged, reassigned from one family or clan to the other. Gayle Rubin writes:

> To enter into a gift exchange as a partner, one must have something to give. If women are for men to dispose of, they are in no position to give themselves away . . . women can't give their daughters to men, because they do not have the same rights in their daughters that their male kin have, rights of bestowal (although *not* of ownership).[19]

Rubin locates gendered oppression in the traffic in women that marks kinship systems, rather than in the traffic in merchandise or products.[20] Thus, rather than just the cold and unfeeling market, it is also family and kinship—social institutions that ostensibly lie outside crass commercialism—that engenders women's subordination. Authentic egalitarianism has not been a part of that earlier form of gift exchange, and to bemoan its loss is nostalgia for a less than ideal past.

Surrogacy has to be located in the entrenched gender and racialized ideologies prevalent in producing *and* consuming societies. Whereas women were exchanged as gifts through the transfer of their intimate, physical, and caring labors from their natal homes to their marital homes, today they themselves possess the right to sell their own labors on reproductive markets. That is, they control the ability to make the decision to commodify their intimate labors. Rather than deeming surrogacy as the inauguration of unprecedented alienation that causes anomie—because a gift has been converted into a commodity—it is perhaps more useful to think through who controls the right to convert a gift into a commodity, and what the marketization of intimate life means. These working-class women in Bangalore undoubtedly have more power than ever before to control their own reproductive destinies, to utilize, commodify or not in ways they want, and to enter reproductive markets. But what does that mean? Are these grand gestures of autonomy, freedom, and choice to do with one's body as one wishes?

The women in Bangalore explained that they became surrogate mothers not simply to put a roof over their heads or food on the table, because they already had that. They were not destitute. But they were desperate. It is this desperation that warrants scrutiny. Though some women engaged in surrogacy for their children's well-being, as had Indirani and Kavita, other women engaged in surrogacy in order to care for aging parents or in-laws, as had Prabha. They were devoted to them, and took it upon themselves to provide for their wants and needs. Or others, like Salma and Chitra, sought to build their own self-worth through the possession of money. Because they were women they had little social power and very little room for maneuver within their marital households. They recognized the disadvantages that accrued to them because of their gender identities—girl children were not preferred; sexual harassment at the workplace was rampant; sexual abuse of their young daughters a real threat; husbands held them in disregard; their gendered labor received little or no social recognition and appreciation; and finally, some of the women's marital extended families held them in contempt, seeing them as burdens rather than as loving, contributing members of the family. A more complicated picture of gender ideologies, household work, and caring, loving familial labor replaces the much-circulated storyline of frantically poor surrogate mothers who pursue reproductive assembly line work solely for the sake of their children. In the place of such a narrative another emerges, where women are working their networks and vending their reproductive abilities and intimate caring in order to achieve social worth in their worlds. As Dr. Gunasheela had asserted, women were indeed empowered through the control of money; but this empowerment has to be located in the larger sociopolitical context.

While Hochschild maintains that money corrupts social relationships, sociologist Viviana Zelizer documents how social life transforms the meaning of money.[21] A rupee or a dollar is not the same as another rupee or dollar. Depending on who earns it and how it is earned, that money may get directed to specific uses. Women and men channel or earmark money for specific needs within their families and communities. A mother's earnings may go toward her children's education whereas the father's earnings may be diverted to paying the rent and putting food on the table. Rather than money eroding social life, as Arlie Hochschild is wont to believe, the entry of money subtly alters but more often, as I show, *solidifies* social relationships and gender roles. Suma, Indirani, and Kavita continued their motherly duties and struggled to make their children's lives better. Prabha and Vijaya extended their feminine, nurturing activities to include underage brothers, elderly mothers, and aging in-laws. Salma, Nagu, and Chitra did not change the fact that women accrue *bele* or social value by controlling money; they earned money so that they could accumulate *bele*.

As feminist scholar Deniz Kandiyoti (1988) eloquently says, women strategize within a set of concrete constraints that reveal the contours of what she terms the "patriarchal bargain" of that society. Prevalent gender norms in their societies call for specific overt and covert strategies in order to not just navigate, but also maximize, their individual status within their kin networks. Kandiyoti continues, "[P]atriarchal bargains exert a powerful influence" on gendered subjectivities, and "they influence both the potential for and specific forms of women's active or passive resistance in the face of their oppression."[22] The money Bangalore's surrogate mothers made by selling their reproductive services circulated through many of the same old gendered gridlines that demarcated their social worlds. Though women controlled decision-making processes regarding their bodies, they were unable to fundamentally alter prevailing gender or class ideologies. Their participation in Bangalore's reproductive assembly lines simply provided them more negotiability within established social norms.

Yet these women had not received wages for pregnancy before. How, then, do they make sense of pregnancy as wage employment? The story of how the women understand the receipt of wages for pregnancy, I maintain, has to be anchored to their personal histories as wage workers, in this case, garment workers. But along with wage exchange, the women also viewed surrogacy in light of another kind of exchange, and that is, the exchange of babies and children among kith and fictive kin. The next chapter maps how women conceptualize their engagement in surrogacy—as wage labor or as gift—by locating these actions in other kinds of exchange, namely, their employment as garment workers and the prevalent practice of sharing children among extended and immediate families, and an underground market in babies.

PART II

Incorporating Pregnancy and Childbirth into the Market Economy

4

Locating Surrogacy in Child Sharing and Wage Labor

Though surrogacy was new, other forms of exchange in children have a long history among southern Indian families. Stories of children who were raised by kith and kin are part of everyday life, retold again and again in Hindu mythologies, but also practiced quite widely. Almost every Hindu child knows that god Krishna was not raised by his mother, but by her close friend Yashoda.[1] My own father had been given away to his maternal aunt when he was a child. His mother was pregnant with her youngest and eighth child, and my grandfather was sick. My father's maternal aunt stepped in by taking my father, the third-born child, off my grandmother's hands.

The surrogate mothers too related stories of such "child sharing" in their families. For example, surrogate mother Suma's youngest sister was childless, so Suma sent her second-born son to be raised by her sister. Indirani's oldest brother and his wife were childless; a poorer cousin had sent his child to the couple who were now raising the child as their own. These sorts of child sharing were a form of gift giving among adults within extended families. To deal with the challenges of raising large families in difficult circumstances, or to assuage the pain of infertility among loved ones, parents temporarily transferred parental rights in their children to supportive or needy kith and kin, as the case may be. These children who were "gifted," were nurtured by loving aunts and uncles and grew up among their cousins, but they were not estranged from their natal families. The concerned adults maintained thick social ties, their lives interwoven together through kinship networks and through frequent interactions with each other on formal and informal social occasions. In fact, in direct contrast to surrogacy, sharing children signaled deeper and stronger social ties between the two families.[2]

Underground Markets in Babies

However, over the course of my daily sojourns to the garment districts of Bangalore I was confronted with other stories of exchange in babies, in which they were exchanged for money. Along with the seventy surrogate mothers I interviewed, I met nine mothers who had either given away their babies to complete strangers for money or had their newborns stolen from them. I met all these women through Roopa. Growing up in Bangalore, I had heard of hospital staff stealing newborn babies and giving them to middle-class families. It was a common narrative that circulated among Bangalore's working-class women who delivered babies at public hospitals *only* if they had family members who could keep a watchful eye on the infant at all times; I had presumed this was an urban myth.

Rather than babies who mysteriously disappeared in government-run hospitals, all the stories I heard during fieldwork involved public hospital staff who approached the indigent family with requests that they give away the newborn baby to another family who could raise it in far greater affluence than could the birth family. Poverty-stricken women, often because their husbands were sick, alcoholic, or dead, gave up their newborn babies because they needed the money to care for their older children, and could ill-afford yet another child in the household.

Roopa herself was involved two years earlier in the case of a middle-class childless couple who took a newborn baby girl from a mother for a sum of money. "This is common among women who work in *agarbathi* [incense] factories, *akka*," said Roopa. One such person was Saraswati, a thirty-five-year-old *agarbathi* worker and mother of three children. The youngest of three daughters, and raised by her grandparents because her own parents were destitute, she had studied up to the ninth standard in a government school. She was married off at the age of twenty to an alcoholic man. Pregnant with a second child at twenty-four, she had a large loan and desperately needed money to support herself and her toddler son. Her oldest sister arranged for her to give away her newborn baby to a childless couple who lived in the neighboring city of Mysore. Saras-

wati delivered the baby at home, breas
him away in exchange for money. "I st
quently gave birth to a son, now eigh
and then opted for permanent steril
longed for her second son, but he
the three who lived with her and
said, "no one asks you how muc
the question is always this, Ho
think so? No one asks how much mo
dren is a blessed home because it is filled with
Every day I miss that son of mine."

Her alcoholic husband still did not support the family. Instead, h
oldest son, now fourteen, performed odd jobs at various factories so he could earn money for his mother and his younger siblings. "Why don't you ask your husband to leave?" I asked Saraswati. She laughed and replied, "You know how our people are. They say a household with a husband is a fortunate one even when that man is useless."

Nagalaxmi was another such mother. She worked at home making *agarbathis*. She now has two children. She had always believed that her second-born baby died at childbirth, but learned otherwise when she was pregnant the third time around. Her husband confessed that he had colluded with his parents to sell the second baby in order to obtain funds for his mother's medical bills. They had collectively lied to Nagalaxmi and told her that the baby girl had died at childbirth and they did not want her to see the newborn's "dead" body because it would be too traumatic for her. Nagalaxmi could not forgive her husband, yet did not know how to raise her two children without his support. So she stayed with him.

And then there was Usha, the only daughter of a truck driver. Because her father traveled extensively and her mother worried for the safety of her then nine-year-old child, she was sent off to work as a live-in maid for a middle-class family with two children of their own. When Usha turned eighteen her parents arranged her marriage for her, and she was soon pregnant. However, her former employers began making baby because they wanted a child for their own child- who resided in the United States. When the newborn baby e days old her former employers arrived at her home, and baby away from her. Usha and her husband felt they could not t because her father owed the former employers money. She was ply resentful but felt powerless to do anything; and reassured herself y saying that at least her daughter had a life that she herself could never afford. Perhaps this was better for the child.

In this context of illegal markets in babies it is perhaps not surprising that infertility doctors and surrogacy agencies insisted that surrogacy empowered women. If there already was an underground market in babies, how wrong could surrogacy be? At least this way women could make calculated decisions about how to deploy their reproductive capabilities in legally endorsed ways, instead of making last-minute desperate decisions that led to illicit exchanges. Surrounded by stories of baby sharing and selling that occurred in their neighborhoods and within their own families, some women did not see surrogacy as a vastly aberrant social practice. There were already well-established socially endorsed *and* clandestine circulations of children in place, and now they were jumping into the fray themselves.

But more than simply jumping into the fray, some surrogate mothers experienced their labor engagements on reproductive assembly lines as life-affirming. Many mothers constantly contrasted other forms of wage labor to surrogacy. They frequently raised their employment in garment sweatshops as a point of contrast to their employment on reproductive assembly lines. Why did garment sweatshop work loom so large in their imaginations? I would learn from speaking with women who worked in garment sweatshops.

From Garment Sweatshops to Reproductive Assembly Lines

"*Aiyo akka*, we garment workers . . . our lives are hell, hell, hell. And our worlds are destroyed, destroyed, destroyed," declared Lalitha dramatically.[3] It was the end of my first field visit to Bangalore, and I was sitting on the floor with fifteen women garment workers in one of their homes located in a part of the city where garment factories abound and COTW is located. Very early in my research I had learned that almost all the women living in the dormitory had previously been garment workers. Hot on the tracks of postindustrial markets in life, I had unexpectedly found myself back at the doorstep of industrial garment work. Women moved from garment sweatshops to Bangalore's reproduction assembly lines, first selling their eggs and then going into surrogacy.

Most of the surrogate mothers I interviewed had long and intermittent working histories. Some were housewives. Some like Vijaya were employed when they themselves were mere children, from eight to nine years of age, residing as live-in "maids" with middle-class families to take care of children not much older than them. Their life stories revealed that some of the women were engaged in intimate labor since childhood, shifting from child care to surrogacy over their life course. The majority of the surrogate mothers, however, were garment workers. As garment workers they earned $100–150 per month, which was a lot more than what many other working-class women in Bangalore make. Anecdotal information and informal conversations with other researchers suggest that this garment-reproduction nexus is unique to Bangalore. Part of the reason for this is because of the preponderance of women garment workers in the city, which is atypical in India. Whereas in the rest of the country just over 60 percent of garment workers are women, in Bangalore over 80 percent of the workers are women.[4]

Creative Options Trust for Women (COTW) is located in the heart of one of the city's garment neighborhoods. The garment industry has advantages for surrogate mother recruiters because these factories house large numbers of women workers in prime reproductive age. Recruiting agents also have extensive networks among women in their prime fertility who are housewives, salesgirls, or household maids. However, their greatest recruiting success is among garment workers. In the next section I describe Bangalore's garment industry, the chief source of employment for working-class women, to partially understand why surrogacy was a preferred labor option.

Bangalore's Garment Industry

Prior to its rise to global prominence as India's "Silicon Valley," the center of outsourced information technology work from various parts of the world, from 1900 to 1950 textiles dominated Bangalore's industry.[5] From World War II, however, Bangalore's industrial landscape began to change. The Hindustan Machine Tools and Bharat Electronic Ltd. were established in 1952 and 1953, respectively. And by the 1960s the city had solidified its reputation as a research-centered urban area; the Indian Space Research Organization, the Defense Research and Development Organization, and the Central Power Research Institute were all established in various parts of Bangalore. All these large, capital-intensive, state-sponsored public sector initiatives were accompanied by the development of private subsidiary factories that produced machine parts, tools, and plastic goods. In 1983 there were 9,959 registered small-scale industries in the city; in the next decade small industries increased by almost three times to 26,534 registered units. Alongside, the informal sector workforce grew in the city. In 1971 55.25 percent of Bangalore's workforce was in the informal sector; by 1991 this had grown to 72 percent.[6]

A large part of this growth was abetted by the government's small-scale industries' policy that provided subsidies for small, privately owned units. In addition, in 1966 the Karnataka Industrial Areas Development Board established the Peenya industrial district on the outskirts of the city through land acquisitions acts, to cater to the needs of small-scale industries. Currently, almost 70 percent of the city's garment units are located in this industrial belt that runs from the west of the city all the way down to its southern end.[7] Today, Bangalore's garment industry comprises numerous small and large firms such as Arvind Mills, which

is the world's fourth largest exporter of denim
Marks & Spencer, Levis, Tommy Hilfiger, ar
in comparison to Gokaldas Exports. Amo
concerns to be established in Bangalore
owns 46 factories in and around Banga
ployees. Gokaldas counts among its c
crombie and Fitch, Levi's, Dockers, H&M, and

Bangalore, then, is not just India's Silicon Valley bu
Galli.[9] Just as ubiquitous as the male software engineer is the w
garment worker rushing every morning, lunch bag in hand, to board the bus to get to a sweatshop. Investigations by the New Trade Union Initiative (NTUI) show that Bangalore has the most feminized garment workforce in the country; 84 percent of the garment workers are women and 81 percent of the workers are below thirty years of age.[10] A vast majority of these workers have completed middle school, and 60 percent belong to the Vokkaliga Gowda community and other dominant castes such as the Gownder, who originate in the neighboring state of Tamil Nadu.[11] Research also shows that Bangalore's women garment workers put in over sixteen hours of work a day at the factory and at home. Their most time-consuming chores outside the factory are laundry, cooking, child care, and commuting to work.[12]

While I have no data on the health of garment workers in Bangalore, research in Dhaka's garment factories shows that workers had headaches, chest pain, ear and eye pain, general anemia, gastritis, nausea, cough, cold and other forms of respiratory difficulties, urinary tract infections (UTIs), and reproductive health problems. Nearly 18 percent of the Bangladeshi women surveyed had suffered from UTIs the previous month. Of these, 40 percent said they had had UTIs for almost an entire month. Tellingly, the supervisors, almost all men, suffered the least from illnesses.[13] In addition, workers had accidents such as pierced or crushed fingers, and electrical shocks due to faulty wiring. Women made 41 percent less money than their male colleagues. On average, the workers surveyed in Dhaka said they put in twelve-hour days at the nd there was no provision for paid leave. The Dhaka research that the average length of a garment worker's working life is four s. Only 14 percent of the workers had worked continuously for over ven years, and 26 percent of the women surveyed said they were planning to quit soon.[14]

Garment work can be brutalizing largely because of the short, intense production cycles driven by demand from retailers such as Gap or H&M who are themselves obliged to stock their shelves for the upcoming fashion season. The first time I met with fifteen garment workers I learned that they were expected to meet inordinately high production quotas. If the women were unable to meet their quotas they were verbally abused in order to get them to work faster. The women said they did not want to draw the supervisors' attention—almost all of them men—upon themselves because these men castigated them in sexual terms, and sometimes groped them sexually to humiliate them in front of their coworkers. To avoid the rampant sexual harassment women faced on the shop floor, some women (like Roopa) did piecework at home for small factories. At the factory, however, the women worked continuously without taking bathroom breaks. Many new initiates to garment work did not take water bottles with them or drink water over the course of their workday because this created the urge to use the restroom more frequently. The only time most of the garment workers used the restrooms was during the midday forty-five-minute lunch break, and upon completion of work at 6:00 p.m. The women complained that they were prone to urinary tract infections when working in the factory.

Many garment workers in Bangalore noted that the production quotas were set at such high levels that they stayed after hours to catch up on work. But they were never paid overtime wages. The supervisors reasoned that after-hours work made up for inefficiently used time during the workday and did not deserve any compensation. The women said that their husbands and in-laws expressed disapproval when they worked after hours; not only was housework not completed, but they did not receive any pay either. When their paychecks did not reflect their overtime work, their husbands and in-laws wondered whether the women were really at the factory or they were having an extramarital affair. As a result the women reported that they felt degraded at work by their supervisors and at home by castigating family members.

Sweatshop Labor, Women, and Waste

In her study of *maquiladoras*, geographer Melissa Wright (2006) describes the myth of the disposable Third World woman.[15] Because of the long work hours and the repetitive work involved, women workers in sweatshops either burn out or their health deteriorates. Over time they are unable to sustain their productivity and are fired. They become disposable byproducts of the industrial process who are replaced with new workers. Yet when women burn out, fall sick, or have other household duties to attend to and quit work, instead of criticizing the brutalizing work processes, factory supervisors and employers maintain that they have no interest in a career. Their biological destinies as mothers and devotion to family, the employers insist, lead to a lack of corporate loyalty. Thus, high turnover rates among women are posited as *their* choice rather than poor working conditions or low pay. Wright (2006) observes that precisely because they are disposable, working-class women add tremendous value to the production process. Companies from all over the world seek out these disposable women's labor in free trade zones in order to optimize their profits.

In Bangalore's garment factories, women constantly shift from being valuable workers to becoming waste. When a woman is healthy she produces value for the firm; but when she has burned out, fallen sick, become pregnant, or has to take care of children or older members of the family she loses her value as a worker. She is dismissed and replaced with a new worker. Once she recovers her health or manages to take care of her family chores efficiently, she cycles back into the factories again, this time miraculously having regained her value for the industrial process. The women I interviewed strive against the conditions in factories and at home that leave them physically and emotionally exhausted. With few exceptions, their working lives in the factories are over by the time they reach their mid-thirties.

Hope on Reproductive Assembly Lines

Many of the surrogate mothers I met stopped working in garment factories when they burned out. They cycled back in again upon recovering their health because they needed the wages. Over time they felt used up, their physical and emotional health compromised, and their lives slowly destroyed. However, they needed to pay the rent, put food on the table, and educate their children so they could hopefully escape a life of precarity.[16] Under these circumstances Bangalore's reproduction industry offered hope.

Suma avoided garment work altogether because she had witnessed her mother's, maternal aunts', and older sister's lives as garment workers. She stayed home with her two sons who were below the ages of eight. "But I need money," she told me. "For us, surrogacy is a boon." When I met her again in December 2011 Suma was receiving hormonal injections in order to be a surrogate mother the second time around. She knew failure rates for in vitro fertilizations were high and hoped for a positive result.

Time and again the women indicated that even as they were converted to waste in the garment factories, the emerging trade in reproduction allowed them to sell their eggs and receive wages for pregnancy and childbirth. Thus the women moved from production to reproduction assembly lines, embracing egg "donation" and subsequently surrogacy. The emergent commodification of life allowed them to harvest wages from aspects of their lives that had remained outside the market. When I expressed my concerns about repeated hormonally induced hyper-stimulation of ovaries and uteri, many of the surrogate mothers nonchalantly shrugged. None of them had witnessed others developing complications through these highly invasive medical procedures. They indicated that their priority was to find a way out of their precarious economic conditions. Negative health consequences were secondary and they would deal with complications if and when they arose. Other forms of employment in Bangalore, such as cleaning homes, working as cooks, or caring for middle-class children and the elderly, while affording stable wages, did not give the women a lump sum of U.S. $4,000 as did surrogacy, which could be invested in different economic endeavors. As Nagu had eloquently emphasized, even men could not earn such wages. It was only through their unique biological capacities as women that they could earn $4,000, gifting extended families with new opportunities, which greatly increased their social standing and strengthened their hands in familial decision-making processes.

Empowerment through Surrogacy

There is a long history of published scholarship on how commodified caring causes estrangement in care workers.[17] However, in spite of the exploitation that was apparent to them, the women derived far more meaning from selling their eggs and surrogacy than they did under the industrial labor disciplinary regimes of the garment factory. When I first arrived at COTW, I was dismayed to see that the women were sequestered away from their families in women-only dormitories. Though family members visited and sometimes young children lived with their mothers, the women were isolated from their own homes and neighborhoods. Mr. Shetty, the proprietor of COTW, explained that the surrogate mothers' sequestration in dormitories was necessary because it afforded them privacy. Separated from disapproving neighbors and relatives, they could return home after having delivered the babies and no one would know that they had engaged in surrogacy. It was also easier to monitor the women's health in dormitories. The COTW staff found it simpler to coordinate schedules and take various surrogate mothers for their regular prenatal visits with doctors and laboratories where they underwent blood tests, ultrasounds, and other such procedures. Finally, the intended parents felt reassured that the surrogate mothers were housed in safe, clean conditions and ate good, balanced diets.

The mothers complained about the surrogacy dormitory. For example, when they first arrived, Mr. Shetty told the women they could ask the kitchen staff to cook any food they wanted because he wanted to fulfill all the food cravings they'd have as pregnant women. Yet he demurred when they asked for specific foods. He worried that not everyone would eat that food and the kitchen staff would be overworked if every surrogate mother resident was to make dietary demands. The surrogate mothers reserved their greatest derision for Preeti, the dorm manager and Mr. Shetty's lover. She often remarked that the surrogate mothers did not have the economic means to put food on their own tables; what would they know about good or bad food? They would have to make do with what was served. The resident mothers maintained that the ingredients used and the quality of food tended to be substandard.

Yet in spite of their complaints, the women found the dormitory to be a curiously liberating place. Indirani explained that she had felt physically and emotionally exhausted when she worked as a tailor in the garment factory and then returned home to clean, cook, and take care of her family. But when she got pregnant for surrogacy, Indirani stayed away from her family in the COTW dormitory. At first she missed her family, often wondering what her children were doing. Was her mother-in-law taking care of them? "I was surrounded by strangers," she recalled. But soon she began to like the dormitory. She did not have to wake up by 5:00 a.m. to prepare meals for the family, pack lunches for everyone, drop the children off at the bus stop so they could get to school, and then get onto the bus herself to get to the garment factory. Instead, she slept in and was served breakfast when she wanted. She had no household obligations and no one made demands on her time and emotions. Surrogacy afforded her the luxury of being served by others. Indirani explained she could not remember a time in her life when she had felt so liberated from all responsibilities.

Through the surrogacy process, many women told me, they had lost a baby forever but gained sisters for life. They came to recognize that they had more in common with other mothers in the dormitory than with female family members or friends in their neighborhoods. While surrogacy is often seen as a loss to surrogate mothers because they lose the babies they birth, the mothers themselves talked about the gains they had made because of the deeply meaningful, lifelong friendships they established with other women.

"But don't the closed circuit cameras bother you?" I persisted. Walking into the dormitory the first time, I had felt these cameras' invasive presence creating an atmosphere of what felt like a total institution wherein the women were watched constantly in order to supervise every possible infraction. Most of the women said the cameras did not bother them, and often they did not even register the cameras' presence. I realized that they were accustomed to surveillance in their everyday lives. Living under the gaze of relatives and inquisitive neighbors, and housed in one- or two-room homes where it was common for six to eight households to share a bathroom, notions of privacy were relative. Moreover, surveillance at the dormitory was benign compared to the surveillance and punishment meted out for supposed infractions on the garment shop floor, where long conversations, taking a few minutes of rest, or going on bathroom breaks were all curtailed. By comparison, surveillance at COTW, designed to find out whether the women were having sex with their menfolk when they visited the facilities, seemed banal.

A few mothers used the term "*punya*" to describe their work as surrogate mothers; that is, they had the good fortune to accomplish so much through their engagement in mere wage labor. One surrogate mother said that nothing she had accomplished as a wage worker had produced so much social value as that surrogated baby. While many see surrogacy as immoral and surrogate mothers as unethical women who are "baby sellers," the mothers themselves posited their actions as ethically unimpeachable. They contrasted the labor processes involved in surrogacy to garment production. In the garment factory they felt degraded because they were sexually harassed and humiliated by their male shop floor supervisors. And upon returning home, especially on days when they worked overtime but did not receive any overtime pay, their husbands and in-laws cast aspersions on their sexual morality, wondering if they were engaging in extramarital affairs. Their sexual discipline and their personal character under question, working on the garment production line was both physically and emotionally debilitating.

On the other hand, Bangalore's reproduction industry allowed them to be moral workers. At the dormitory they resided in a women's-only space and abstained from sex with even their husbands. They made babies without engaging in sex. By birthing these babies they contributed to the continuation of familial (patriarchal) lineages. Indirani was especially eloquent: she said that through surrogacy she had built a nuclear family unit and fulfilled one infertile woman's desire to be a mother. In the process she had simultaneously attempted to secure the future of her own nuclear family unit and her own happiness. Indirani contrasted the social value of producing babies to producing garments. She said, "Garments? You wear your shirt a few months and you throw it away. But I make you a baby? You keep that for life. I have made something so much bigger than anything I could ever make in the factory."

Indirani and the other mothers did not necessarily see selling eggs or surrogacy as benign processes. Nor did they misread their exploitation. However, given their life options, they believed that Bangalore's reproduction industry afforded them greater control over their emotional, financial, and sexual lives. But crucially, surrogacy was a profoundly creative form of wage employment that allowed women to assert their moral worth. Birthing babies was far more meaningful than producing garments, and because of that women found their involvement on reproductive assembly lines to be life-affirming and profound. Their participation in markets in life, in spite of deepened commodification, was also a peculiarly meaningful experience.

Precarious Work, Precarious Lives

Descriptions of late capitalism map a shift from Fordist methods of production dominated by blue collar jobs to post-Fordism with the rise of service jobs and information technologies. From being immersed in the world of material labor where production involved the making of shirts, car parts, and such, workers now engage in immaterial labor in order to deliver services. I show that not only do industrial and postindustrial workplaces occupy the exact same locales, but they also employ the exact same people. Working-class women in Bangalore transfer their labor from producing garments to the reproduction trade, and back again.

Insecure conditions in one facet of production create and sustain labor markets in others. The vagaries of the market and the economic risks inherent in garment production are systematically displaced from big retailers onto production units that dot various parts of the Third World. These risks are in turn transferred onto individual workers who take on uncertain work, long hours, and hazardous working conditions to make discounted garments that saturate retail stores. The instability of work on the garment shop floor in Bangalore is driven by the cycle of global demands, and the less than ideal working conditions are driven by production deadlines set through local firms' contracts with apparel retailers such as Gap. For garment workers in Bangalore, life is precarious. And precariousness changes the way people organize their lives.[18]

Feminist health organizations such as SAMA based in New Delhi, India, rightfully criticize commercial surrogacy. Along with bioethicists, they describe the reproduction industry as prioritizing the profit motive at the expense of surrogate mothers.[19] I agree with these criticisms, but complicate the narrative by listening to what the mothers say, *not* about their destitution, but about their precarious working lives. Many women, although they mourned the loss of the babies they carried in their bodies, curiously posited surrogacy as a process that empowered them. How are we to make sense of the fact that massive hormonal infusions into the body, long periods of sequestration from their families, and caesarian sections scheduled to deliver babies preterm, are all posited as life-affirming acts? I argue that the conversion of the alienation and pain involved in market pregnancies into empowerment can only be understood within the context of the surrogate mothers' working lives and social worlds. The surrogate mothers were engaged in complex maneuvering; they complied with the gendered discipline and even risky conditions imposed by reproductive market agents in order to negotiate relatively powerful positions for themselves within their households. They submitted to the manipulations of marketplace patriarchy in order to recast familial patriarchy. If they were destroyed by garment sweatshops, then surrogacy became a way by which they attempted to create new worlds.

5

Babies as Commodities

In October 2011 *the New York Times* wrote about a twenty-nine-year-old domestic worker in Delhi named Manju who, when approached by a surrogacy recruiter, was tempted because she could make a lot of money. She said, "Risks? What risks? Any fool can have a baby, it takes a smart woman to get paid for it."[1] Many of the surrogate mothers I met believed that they were, like Manju, smart women because they were getting paid for something they had previously done for free. Even those who regretted surrendering the babies appreciated the earnings through surrogacy. But how did they make sense of the conversion of what had seemed like an unalienable life experience to an alienable form of employment for which they received wages? In this chapter I revisit Indirani and her sisters, who maintained that they wanted surrogacy to remain a commercial transaction and by extension, tacitly acknowledged that the baby was a commodity over whom they *wanted* no rights.

Surrogacy as Wage Labor

I was having lunch with Indirani at her home, with her sisters Kavita and Prabha, and their friends Kala and Suma. The women laughingly reminisced about the bad meals in the dormitory. But they also they talked about all the fun they had had at the dormitory, including going to the beauty parlor together to get their eyebrows plucked, limbs waxed, and facials done. Right after that they had gone to a studio to have professional photographs taken of themselves; they proudly showed me these photographs. They also fondly recalled the time they'd gone to a weavers' cooperative together to buy themselves silk saris. And they reminisced about the time Indirani's recipients[2] would bring treats, different kinds of fruit and foods for her. They brought enough so that she could share with the other residents. Indirani turned to me, recalling: "My recipients were a Tamil couple who lived in the United States and spoke only English, madam. Their mother spoke Tamil but I speak better Kannada than Tamil. What to do? Conversations were hard." From Indirani's descriptions it became apparent that her recipients worked hard to honor her efforts. Late in her pregnancy they conducted a *srimantha* for her, which is a South Indian ritual performed to honor the pregnant woman, celebrate her fertility, and seek divine blessings for the safe birth of a healthy baby. All the resident surrogate mothers and the staff feasted on extravagantly prepared food provided by Indirani's recipients. They made sure they included all her favorite dishes in the menu for the day. As is customary she received a silk sari and a small gold necklace.[3] Amidst discussions of the food they ate and the fun they had, however, Indirani added that rather than having wasted their money on what amounted to conspicuous consumption, she wished the recipients had just given her hard cash. In place of the *srimantha* meant to honor her, she would rather have had the cash the recipients had spent on it.

Indirani's recipients had sincerely attempted to move pregnancy from being alienated labor to socially meaningful work; the intended mother and her mother spent considerable time every week with Indirani, they brought her and her friends fruit and foods, and finally, by performing a *srimantha* they attempted to show their reverence for her considerable efforts. But Indirani was not interested in translating wage labor into something outside the market. Speaking with her, it seemed that from her perspective, pregnancy in surrogacy really was simply a labor process for which she wanted only wages. As she noted earlier, she did not feel any attachment to the twins she had surrogated. The babies, if anyone were to hear her, were indeed commodities exchanged for wage labor.

Though not a surrogate mother yet, her younger sister Kavita held a different perspective. She said:

> Those recipients too struggle for a baby. They pray to god. Similarly, we surrogates pray for strength to give up that baby. I have had three cancelations [failed surrogacy attempts] and don't know how it is to give up a baby. But I know I will cry. I love babies. I feel that if the babies come to know us, they will never accept the recipients as their parents. They will always love us more. But, as a single mother of three children I need money. I will close my heart[4] to that baby and keep my focus on those three children who depend on me. My love and duty is toward them. That is why I'm doing this.

Kavita added that a fair wage for surrogacy would be at least $6,000.

Kala, Kavita's best friend, was twenty-six years old and Gownder by caste. She had studied up to middle school. She grew up in Bangalore as the oldest child of three under the watchful eyes of her flower vendor mother, and her father who worked as a car mechanic. She was married off at the age of nineteen to a man who was a weaver of silk saris. However, he had fallen sick and she had begun working as a garment worker over the past year. Her mother-in-law stayed at home with them, and her father-in-law worked as a security guard for a wealthy family. The household earnings were around $250, but that was not enough to cover expenses. Kala had to provide for a five-year-old son and a three-year-old daughter. She had donated her eggs twice over the past two years but $550 of her loans remained unpaid. Kavita had received $50 both times as a commission from COTW for having recruited Kala; but she did not take any *bakshish* from Kala. Kala now wanted to become a surrogate mother. She had had a failed surrogacy pregnancy seven months earlier and was again receiving hormones in preparation for implantation, which was scheduled for the following week.

She told me about the time of her failed surrogacy attempt. There was no fetal heart beat four months into her pregnancy and they had to "clean" her, she said. Kala asked rhetorically, "Do you know how much it hurts?" I nodded, assuming that the loss of fetal life was painful; instead she went in a different direction:

> We have missed work. We have lost wages. We have left our own little children. It is not as if my mother-in-law is getting any younger. Taking care of my children was very hard on her. . . . [Surrogacy] is a burden on the entire household. It is not easy. And on top of that our bodies have to endure such *himse*.[5] We have all these painful injections and scans [transvaginal ultrasounds]. After all this, imagine how I felt when I miscarried in my fourth month. For all that effort and pain I received nothing. It was a loss for me financially.

Surrogate mothers were legally entitled to partial wages if they miscarried. Many of my intended parent interviewees spoke of how surrogacy in India might be estimated at $34,000 to $36,000 for singleton babies, but in truth the costs were higher because this did not cover the expenses of "canceled" cycles, which could run as high as $20,000. If a surrogacy attempt failed either because the embryos were not viable to begin with, the embryos did not implant, or the surrogate mother miscarried, the intended parents were billed for the doctors' and various technologists' efforts, and for the surrogate mother's exertions.[6]

By Indian law surrogate mothers who miscarry are entitled to partial wages as compensation for missed days of paid employment and lost wages, and for their efforts in being hyper-stimulated with hormonal shots and transvaginal ultrasounds. Moreover, the mothers have also spent considerable amounts of money in making arrangements for child care when they are in dormitories. Some of them take on loans in order to fund the expenses they incur during surrogacy. A failed surrogacy attempt, then, is not just physical hardship but also a financial loss.

None of the Bangalore surrogate mother interviewees knew they were entitled to partial compensation. They explained that Mr. Shetty routinely "gifted" them $100 for the pain of their failed pregnancies. But he would subtract this amount from the $4,000 they earned in their subsequent, and eventually successful attempts at surrogacy. Many of the seventy women I met, with the exception of Pushpa, had tried again and again until they had successful pregnancies, and Mr. Shetty always recovered his $100 "gift." The women were incentivized to try surrogacy again and again in order to recover some of their losses.[7]

I asked Kala whether she'd want to hold the baby she'd give birth to, and she replied, "What is the point of seeing a baby who will never be in my life? As a mother of two children, a sick husband, and an aging mother-in-law I have enough problems. I'd rather have more money because I have all these dependents."

"But won't you feel bad giving up this baby?" I persisted. "The baby had moved in you, woken you up in the mornings, or kicked that much harder after you've had your cup of . . . ?" Indirani forcefully cut me short.

> No. Right from the beginning you need to convince yourself that this baby is not yours. Right from the beginning, tell your mind. And when you talk to others always refer to this as someone else's baby. This is my advice to everyone. Do not grow to desire (*aase*) the baby. . . . In my mind I have no feelings, madam. For my own children I struggle hard enough. Why would I need more children in my life? Loving children is a burden. I don't want any contact with the babies, the twins I birthed. One should not have feelings. I was the one who gave Suma courage when she was devastated about giving up the baby. . . . She'd cry and I'd reprimand her . . . that she has sons. Why have you come here? I asked. To cope with your difficulties, to repay your loans, or have you come here to make more difficulties for yourself? . . . If there was no egg donation or surrogacy, then what would we do to earn that kind of money?

The potential for earning a lump sum of $4,000 seemed promising, given that their households netted around $200 to $250 per month. This opportunity was available to them only because of their capacity to get pregnant, grow life within their bodies, and birth babies. Their gendered bodies, socially and economically undervalued in workplaces such as garment factories, were precisely the site of creation, commodification, and generation of surplus value. However, their earnings from surrogacy dissipated in a matter of months. They came to understand that their labor was worth more than $4,000.

Most intended parents in Bangalore were billed up to $8,000 to $10,000 per baby for the surrogate mothers' services. Or they paid up to $15,000 for twins. Media sources report that surrogate mothers received up to $8,000 in places like Anand, Gujarat, but almost all the mothers in Bangalore earned only $4,000 whether they had carried singletons or twins. Some mothers said they knew that Mr. Shetty charged clients $360 per month toward housing surrogate mothers, yet he paid the women $60 per month (which was included in the $4,000 wages they received). They acknowledged that he incurred expenses in housing, providing food, taking the women to their various appointments, and maintaining recruiting agents and staff to run COTW, but surely all this did not cost $300 per woman? They were aware that Mr. Shetty's profit margins were large. The surrogate mothers believed they should receive anywhere from $6,000 to $8,000 for their work. Why did women get paid so little for their considerable efforts?

Sociologist Paula England says that jobs, including ones such as surrogacy, have two kinds of compensation; one is pecuniary, and the other non-pecuniary, that is, good work conditions compensate for lower wages. Some employers and scholars believe that women earn less than men because they "care more about non-pecuniary rewards (such as avoiding physical danger or having mother-friendly work conditions) than men," and are willing to "trade off earnings for amenities by choosing safer, more mother-friendly jobs,"[8] which allow women to work around family obligations. However, Paula England says there is no empirical evidence to support this belief. In the case of surrogacy too, this is not true; medical interventions and surgeries make surrogacy a risk-laden work process. And surrogacy is not a mother-friendly job either, because women are kept sequestered in dormitories for months on end, away from their children and gendered household responsibilities. Instead of the nonpecuniary aspects to jobs that are used to justify low wages, Paula England clarifies that because women are devalued in sexist societies, their work is devalued too. These devaluations get solidified in the labor market. She expands:

> Cultural ideas deprecate work done by women, and cultural beliefs lead to cognitive errors in which decision makers underestimate the contribution of female jobs. . . . [O]nce wage scales are set up, the disparities are perpetuated by organizational inertia in the form of using past wages within the organization to set present wages or the use of market surveys of wages in other firms to set jobs' pay levels. That is, wage scales get "institutionalized."[9]

Listening to the mothers, it was apparent that the considerable intellectual, mental, and emotional energy that went into converting pregnancy from a meaningful, nonalienable event to wage labor was *assumed* to be a given, rather than explicitly recognized and compensated. Surrogacy agencies, infertility doctors, and intended parents implicitly assumed that working-class women did not have to struggle to convert their vulnerable bodies into the industrial machines that were required for Bangalore's reproduction assembly lines. Instead, women's bodies were already things or automatons meant for technological interventions, which required no real effort by the mothers. It was bad enough that these sacrifices were not remunerated, but the fact that these forms of renunciation and subsequent suffering were not even acknowledged by doctors and some intended parents was deeply hurtful to the mothers.

The Baby as Commodity

One thread of the literature on assisted reproductive technologies and surrogacy explicitly tackles head on the commodification of pregnancy and birth.[10] Now president of Barnard College, Debora Spar (2006) notes, "[W]e don't like to think of children as economic objects. They are products, we insist, of love, not money; of an intimate creation that exists far beyond the reach of any market impulse." Yet recent innovations in medical technology and business organization have "created a market for babies, a market in which parents choose traits, clinics woo clients, and specialized providers earn millions of dollars a year."[11] Revenues from fertility treatments in the United States have grown from $41 million in 1986 to nearly $3 billion in 2002. In her book aptly titled *The Baby Business*, which maps the trade in infertility services and perhaps even babies in adoption, Spar states that the defining aspects of the baby trade are motivated by parental devotion, and thus "virtually all aspects of the baby trade . . . are technical or social ways for parents to acquire children whom they will subsequently rear and love."[12] Because of what babies mean, this market does not "necessarily work like the market for pumpkins or mortgages," maintains Spar. Prices are not flexible, varying by demand or supply, and more importantly, "the very idea of property rights—the core of most modern markets—remains either ambiguous or contested," as it should be with regard to children.[13]

The problem for Debora Spar is not that there is a market in children, but that it is fragmented because various baby procurement procedures such as adoption, fertility treatment, and surrogacy all operate independently of each other. As a result, the valuation of labor, pricing, and such varies widely. In order to make the baby market work effectively, Spar recommends that the business be armed with all the necessary accouterments, including "a semblance of property rights, some common definitions, and a framework that applies across its disparate parts."[14]

While Debora Spar's concern is market fragmentation, legal scholar Naomi Cahn (2009) takes on the fragmentation of legal regulations governing the commerce in children. Laws regarding gamete "donation" vary from those dealing with the determination of parentage; and the laws governing children's rights to learn about their genetic origins often conflict with donors' privacy rights. As a result, Naomi Cahn says the legal regulation of the infertility industry is *ad hoc*, with the wheel being reinvented with every case of conflict that comes to litigation. As a remedy she proposes that legal reform be directed at developing a rigorous, coherent approach that "allocates regulatory responsibility among the federal and state governments, and industry groups."[15] The overall implication is that by regulating the industry, the market can operate with greater clarity, which is a more equitable arrangement because all individuals enter into transactions with coherent understandings of the processes, meanings, and terms governing the reproduction trade.

In contrast to the business and legal models proposed by Debora Spar and Naomi Cohn, respectively, sociologist Amrita Pande (2009) too looks at the commerce of baby production but from the perspective of the surrogate mothers. In her ethnography of surrogate mothers in Anand, Gujarat, Amrita Pande explains that these women are similar to factory workers but are simultaneously caring mothers who are produced through counseling, contractual agreements that force them to surrender the babies born to them, and by installing them for months on end—separating them from their own social worlds—in dormitories with other surrogate mothers like themselves. She calls surrogate mothers "mother workers."[16] Through regimens of activities coordinated according to time schedules over the course of the day, week, and months during their stay in the dormitory, industrial discipline is inculcated in the women, which the infertility clinic harnesses to accumulate surplus value.

Amrita Pande is most closely aligned with geographers and sociologists who draw on Karl Polanyi's masterly treatise, *The Great Transformation* (1944), on how markets first developed. Polanyi notes that land, labor, and money may be exchanged on the market for rent, wages, and interest, but they are fictive commodities because they were *not* produced for the market. They come to be incorporated for exchange purposes in a market society through the suppression of their social value. Goods or products are the only true commodity because in market economies, they are made solely for the purposes of exchange and profit. Extending Polanyi's argument, then, one could say that the baby is the only true commodity because the sole purpose of the entire transnational surrogacy industry is to produce that one person whose existence and exchange from birth mother to parents is mediated through money.

Debora Spar (2006), however, sits on the fence on whether the baby is a commodity. What exactly is being traded, she asks rhetorically, "Is it babies, or health, or happiness or genes? Is it children or families; bits of protoplasm or the prospect of life?"[17] To call the child a commodity would be to establish property rights over an individual, and Spar is reluctant to go in that direction. Instead, she says the money exchanged in surrogacy is for the *services* rendered in making that baby possible, and not for the baby itself. In Debora Spar's perspective the surrogate mothers are not producers in the sense that egg or sperm donors are; instead, they lease out their wombs to make that baby.[18] They are simply providing rental space in their own bodies. Spar does not want to think of babies as property, yet she sees no contradiction in extending the notion of property to surrogate mothers' bodies, their wombs being alienable and available for rent.

The notion that surrogate mothers simply rent their wombs is widely shared. Transnational surrogacy in India is variously described in the media as the nation's rent-a-womb industry, baby factory, or life factory.[19] These popular sources are not so far off the truth, because the industry and various agents do indeed convert the labor effort in a surrogate pregnancy into a rental relationship. The term used in Kannada to refer to surrogate mothers is indicative; they are called *badige thai*, or "rental" mothers.[20] Tellingly, a surrogate mother is not called *hettha thai*, which loosely translates as "birth" mother; she is always a mother-on-rent.

The problem with the notion of the womb as a rental space is that it is impossible to separate womb from woman, and impossible not to recognize her labor. Marx beautifully draws on the distinction between a honeybee that builds a hive and an architect who designs a building. Marx notes that the bee may be far more skilled in its task, but the architect is far more creative; her work is not simply instinctual as in the bee's effort in building a hive. The architect has truly labored because she draws on her personal history and the larger context, her imagination, and her knowledge of raw materials in order to create that design.[21] Thus, for Marx human labor is infinitely creative, generating in that person knowledge about themselves, their limits and possibilities, and finally, knowledge about the world around them. By doing, that is, sinking their bodies into earthly material, human beings learn about the physical properties of matter such as wood, water, and soil.

Drawing on Marx's distinction, political philosopher Mary O'Brien observes that a woman's reproductive labor is like that of bee *and* an architect. That is, a pregnant woman works on instinct much like the bee, but she also has consciousness like the architect. She remarks:

> [F]emale reproductive consciousness knows that a child will be born, knows what a child is, and speculates in general terms about this child's potential. Yet mother and architect are quite different . . . unlike the architect, her will does not influence the shape of her product. Unlike the bee, she knows that her product, like herself, will have a history. Like the architect, she knows what she is doing; like the bee, she cannot help what she is doing.[22]

Feminist philosopher Nancy Hartsock notes that women's experience in reproduction requires a unity of mind and body far more profound than any wage worker's instrumental activity.[23]

What does it mean, then, to separate babies as singular, unattached life forms who have nothing to do with the surrogate mothers who bear them in wombs that have been converted into alienable property, "leased" for the purposes of growing babies? Are such extreme and multiple levels of estrangement of mother from womb, labor, and baby possible? From an ethical stance, the answer *should* be a resounding no. Yet market practices lead to exactly this kind of alienation of mother from womb, mother from labor, and mother from baby. And the surrogate mothers work very hard to actualize that alienation. In the following section I will discuss the various ways by which surrogate mothers explain the labors involved in surrogacy. They believe that this effort goes unrecognized and they should be adequately compensated.

Calculating Fair Wages for Pregnancy

Sita, a twenty-six-year-old homemaker, had never imagined herself as a wage worker, let alone a surrogate mother. Her husband had a good job; his brother too lived with them and contributed financially to running the household comprising the three adults and two children aged four years and six months, respectively. They lived in a nice rental house and had a car of their own. However, all this changed when Sita's nuclear family was involved in a fatal road accident. Sita's 4 year-old son escaped unscathed. She broke her arm. Her husband sustained life-threatening head injuries, but her six-month-old baby, who had sat on her lap during the ride, was killed instantly. Sita was devastated. When I first met her at the dormitory she kept repeating the story of her baby daughter's death. She showed me the newspaper cutting of the report on their accident, which she kept with her at all times under her bed pillow. She became a surrogate mother in order to pay a part of the $14,000 debt incurred in order to pay her husband's medical bills. She and her husband despaired. Their daughter had passed away in that fatal accident; now, because of surrogacy, they felt like they were selling their own child. By the end of her contract, however, Sita, who was pregnant with twins, had surrendered *two* babies for wages.

Listening to the mothers over the course of the surrogacy it became apparent that the process of commodification is not a given, or an established social truth; instead, it is negotiated by individual women over time, perhaps even before they signed on as surrogate mothers. Sita, whom I met numerous times right from when she lived in the dormitory early in her pregnancy, to a few days after she had delivered the twin babies, exemplified this conversion process of pregnancy to wage labor.

Indirani constantly repeated in various conversations that she had no desire for the twins she surrogated. Her refrain to the other mothers was to think about their own living children whose needs had not been met. Markets in life allowed them to earn large sums of money. Yet most mothers drew attention to the unfairness of the exchange because their wages fell short of the economic, personal, and social costs they had incurred, and the enormity of the sacrifices they and their families had made. The mothers explained the hardships they underwent, which remained unacknowledged and therefore unremunerated.

Unremunerated Familial Labor

Kala was among the most articulate of all the mothers in describing the financial losses that she and her family had sustained in her one failed attempt at surrogacy. Not only had she missed work and wages at the garment factory over the three-and-a-half-month period during which she was hormonally stimulated and implanted with the embryo. In addition her aging mother-in-law had to cook for and take care of her two young children, for which the older woman received no financial compensation. Some husbands were able to balance the additional household tasks along with their employment outside the house if their children were nine or ten years of age because these children took on the absent mother's household responsibilities. But many men with small children were unable or unwilling to do so, and women had to make alternative arrangements for child care. Often they sent the children to their parents' or in-laws' homes. Still others paid friends and neighbors, or depended on these women's generosity to take care of their children. For example, Suma paid a friend $20 every month to house, feed, and take care of her oldest and youngest sons. Her middle son lived with her sister, who bore all his expenses. Thus, not only did they put in their individual labor effort, but their family and friends also expended their energy and emotions, and made sacrifices in order to assist them through surrogacy.

These kinds of familial labor subsidized Bangalore's surrogacy industry. The mothers depended on the goodwill and support of extended kin, neighbors, and friends to provide care and labor for their dependent children so that they could successfully fulfill the terms of their labor contracts that required them to stay in the dorms. These kin and friendship ties were the substance of the women's lives, and because of that they were not burdens. Yet these sorts of demands on others' time, effort, and emotions were substantial, and the mothers felt indebted to their kinswomen and felt they needed to reciprocate in kind in the future.[24]

Pain of Separation from Families

One afternoon I spoke with Selvi, Ganga, Neeta, Chandra, and Kavita in the latter's home. All Kavita's recruitees, the first three had been surrogate mothers together in COTW. Chandra, not yet a surrogate mother, was worried about the extended stay in the dormitory. She said:

> My husband loves the food I cook. This is the taste he has grown accustomed to. . . . To sit with his family—his wife and children—during dinner after a day's work is his greatest happiness. For all of us to be together in the house—it is pure joy! No one likes to eat alone because it is a *sankta* (hardship).[25] Sometimes I invite my friends over too. To have a house full of people fills me with happiness. Now when I go off to the dormitory the house is going to sit empty. My children will stay with my mother, and my husband will be alone at home.

Chandra was currently being prepped for surrogacy and her separation from her family was imminent. She said that her husband wept every evening, imagining what it would be like to be separated from his wife and two children. At these times, she said she caressed his head and comforted him that she would be gone for just nine months. She would return, and they could all be together again. He'd be reassured but then begin to cry again and she would weep too.

As a single mother Kavita said she wanted to stay home with her three children:

> I love my children. . . . I worry about how even my mother will take care of them. I cannot stand the idea of her reprimanding my chil-

> dren or physically punishing them. . . . I'd rather do this [surrogacy] at home. I will not commit any wrongs. I will be exactly as the agency wants me to be.

Many mothers said they worried about their children when they lived in the dormitory. They wondered whether their children ate dinner or breakfast. Did they complete their homework? Did they get to school on time? Were they safe walking to school without their mothers? And they said their children missed them deeply too. The surrogate mothers often remarked on how much weight their children had lost when they were absent from their homes. Their worst fears were realized when their children fell ill. Suma's three-year-old son got very sick with infected sores on his upper body when his mother was at the dormitory. She teared up as she said: "This child has suffered so much. In trying to give a child to another family I almost lost my own."

Being apart from their own young children was especially hard on the surrogate mothers who were in unhappy marriages. Roopa, now separated from her husband, had been a surrogate mother three years earlier when she and her physically abusive husband still lived together. She said she was constantly apprehensive for her then seven-year-old daughter because her husband was an indifferent father. He often came home late and the young child would wait all alone in the dark of the night after having eaten dinner at a neighbor's house. Or worse, he might come home drunk, which could have jeopardized her daughter's safety. Thus, surrogacy, which guaranteed her a lump sum of money she would use to eventually walk out on her abusive husband and lead an independent life with her daughter, also meant that she had to compromise her daughter's well-being for the nine months they were apart. Even though she saw her daughter on weekends, for Roopa nine months was an exceptionally long time to stay away from a seven-year-old, especially from the perspective of the young one who lived under less than ideal conditions at home with an alcoholic and indifferent father. "My child has suffered," said Roopa.

When the children fell sick, if they were young, the staff at the COTW surrogacy dormitory allowed them to come live with their mothers for a few days. The mothers were grateful for these small gestures of kindness, but separations from family, particularly children, were sacrifices that went unrecognized and uncompensated.

The Discomfort and Risks Associated with Contractual Pregnancies

Some surrogate mothers explained that surrogacy entailed *himse*, which means harm, injury, and violence toward the surrogate mothers. This violence was evident through the medical interventions they endured.

While the hormonal injections women undergoing infertility assistance receive in order to hyper-ovulate or thicken the endometrial linings of their uteri have been described as varying from mildly uncomfortable to excruciating, with severe bloating associated with egg retrieval, many surrogate mothers I met did not talk about these procedures as being particularly painful. Only women like Kala and Kavita who had failed surrogacy attempts said the hormonal injections hurt; most others said they felt no fear or pain, or more likely, they'd shrug their shoulders and respond in various ways as Indirani did—they were glad reproductive markets existed because they ostensibly opened the doors to prosperity.

One other aspect of surrogacy the mothers never spoke about was "selective reduction," that is, the selective abortion of fetuses. Because up to four embryos are implanted in women's wombs, more than one of these can develop into a fetus.[26] As a result, doctors commonly practice "selective reduction," where up to three embryos can be aborted depending on the intended parents' requests. Infertility doctors also endorse no more than two fetuses per mother in order to safeguard fetal and maternal health. Potassium chloride is injected into the fetuses selected for "reduction," after which the heart stops and the fetal tissue is reabsorbed into the maternal body. If more than one fetus needs to be eliminated, doctors stagger the procedure over two or so weeks, systematically injecting potassium chloride into one fetus at a time, to protect the remaining fetuses from sudden hormonal fluctuations that can destroy them too. The women are ordered bed rest while doctors serially reduce one, two, or three fetuses over a given period of time. Though none of the women I interviewed spoke of the discomfort of fetal reduction, some intended parent interviewees explained that the surrogate mothers they had contracted with found these reduction procedures exceedingly uncomfortable physically and emotionally.[27]

Almost all the surrogate mothers I interviewed had delivered, or were scheduled to deliver babies, through caesarean surgeries between the thirty-sixth and thirty-eighth weeks of their pregnancies. Though almost all the women, with the exception of one or two cases, had delivered their own one to three children through vaginal births, in order to have complete control over the birthing process and to time the arrival of the babies in accordance to intended parents' schedules, the doctors performed caesarean surgeries on the mothers. The first time I met the surrogate mothers at the dormitory in March 2011 almost all of them were under the misconception that they would deliver the babies through vaginal births. I was the bearer of the bad news that they would undergo major abdominal surgery in order to fulfill the terms of their surrogacy contracts.

Recruiter Sarita, who had accompanied me to COTW, reassured the women that the doctors knew what they were doing. Because these babies were conceived through medical intervention they had to be removed out of the women's wombs through medical intervention. Moreover, she told them, these contractual pregnancies were different from their own because over the course of these pregnancies they did not have sex with their husbands for nine months. Because of sexual inactivity their bodies could not handle vaginal births and they needed caesarians.[28] Sarita encouragingly added that the doctors had performed thousands of caesarian sections over the course of their medical practices. At this point she lifted her *kameez* and pulled the band of her pajamas down to point to the scar across her lower abdomen, indicating that she herself had delivered her daughter through C-section five years before and had suffered no side effects. Sarita assured the mothers that the doctors had nothing to gain from harming them.

Over the course of our subsequent meetings I reiterated the potential risks of caesarian sections. But by then the mothers I had first met had all delivered their babies through C-sections and they believed they had not been harmed. Suma's friend Payal was the only one who said that the spot on her spinal cord where she received her epidural in order to prepare her for caesarian surgery still hurt. But she had not seen a doctor to address this pain because like many of the surrogate mothers I interviewed, she did not receive postnatal care, or postsurgical attention. COTW charged the mothers if they wanted to stay longer in the dormitories to recover from surgery, and they were reluctant to lose their hard earned money. After staying in COTW for two to three days after delivering the babies, the mothers returned home to their own families and the work that awaited them there. The fact that they had been able to get back to their daily routines so quickly after major abdominal surgery proved to them that what they had been told was true; that caesarians were indeed the safest and most convenient method by which to give birth.

More than the pain and discomfort of the hormonal injections, and more than being cut open to deliver the babies, many of the mothers described transvaginal ultrasounds, which they referred to as "scans," as exceedingly humiliating procedures. These women, who have had very little or no access to regular reproductive health care and whose prior pregnancies had been relatively technologically free, were dismayed by the transvaginal ultrasounds they had to undergo as egg donors and surrogate mothers, when doctors checked for follicle, or uterine lining maturity, and the development of the fetus in some cases. They were made to strip naked waist down, lie down on the examination table legs apart, knees bent, and with their feet up in stirrups, while a condom-covered probe was inserted into their vaginas so that the consulting doctor could examine their internal reproductive organs. Mothers viewed such management of their reproductive organs as excessively invasive, far more traumatizing than the caesarian surgeries and the hormonal, ovarian-uterine stimulating injections they received that were associated with long-term health risks. Many women found transvaginal ultrasounds similar to sexual intercourse, because condom-covered phallic-like probes were inserted into their bodies. Suma observed that these procedures were especially traumatic for unmarried egg donors because transvaginal ultrasounds were these sexually inexperienced girls' introduction to vaginal penetration. Some mothers said they had consented to surrogacy, which they assumed was carrying, birthing, and giving up babies while living separately from their own families. But they had *not* consented to the routine instrumental intrusions into their bodies, which felt like a series of sexual assaults.

The mothers described the various forms of *himse* (harm or violence) committed to their bodies, to some of which they had consented and to many others of which they had not. These kinds of bodily intrusions caused physical bodily harm. But more important, from their perspective, was the shame and humiliation they endured, which they felt was grossly underestimated.

The Emotional Labor in Creating Distance from Contractual Babies

Along with these forms of unrecognized and devalued physical hardships, the mothers described the emotional and intellectual labor they performed in their surrogacy contracts. This was especially apparent in the distance they created between themselves and the fetus, positing the yet-to-come baby as an alien being to whom they had no emotional ties.

To be sure, not *all* the surrogate mothers I spoke with felt connected with the fetuses they nurtured in their bodies. This was the mistaken assumption I made in my first set of interviews based on my own life experiences as a mother. My second child, a seven-month-old baby when I first began fieldwork, traveled everywhere with me. He made three trips back and forth to Bangalore and Austin over the course of the year; my baby and I were inseparable. I projected my own feelings of maternal wonder and devoted attachment onto the surrogate mothers.

My acceptance of the connectedness and love pregnant women feel for their imminent babies as a universal truth was grossly a-sociological. Not all women who find themselves pregnant want to birth babies; it is not a leap of faith to claim that those who are accidently pregnant, for example, might be apprehensive and conflicted about becoming mothers. On the other hand, those who *want* to be pregnant are delighted, frequently thinking of even a three-month-old fetus as a baby and eagerly awaiting the birth of that child. Moreover, women say that even with planned pregnancies, they feel differently toward different pregnancies. A woman pregnant for the first time might feel awe and wonder, carefully charting diet and exercise to optimize birthing and neonatal health outcomes. On the other hand, she might feel differently the second time she is pregnant because her circumstances are changed with one child already in her life making caring demands, which might orient her in fundamentally different ways toward her second pregnancy. It is not that she does not want this second pregnancy, but her engagement with it—as a bodily event and life experience—might be radically different from her involvement with her first pregnancy.

The life circumstances of the surrogate mothers affected how they thought about their pregnancies. The forms of labor practice, the devaluation of labor effort on the garment shop floor, and the gradual physical degradation of their bodies, as described in an earlier chapter, had profound effects on their approach to wage work, including pregnancy as a form of effort separable from their minds and bodies, something which could be alienated from their being and sold on the labor market. My assumption that the surrogate mothers felt toward their contractual pregnancies just as they did when pregnant with their own children who lived with them was a mistake. Surrogacy pregnancies felt fundamentally different. To begin with, they knowingly entered into contracts where they received money in return for babies *meant to be given away* at birth. The mothers were counseled to that effect even before they signed their surrogacy contracts, and they approached these contractual pregnancies differently even before they got pregnant. Additionally, their pregnancy in surrogacy was facilitated by substantial medical interventions, which was not the case with their earlier pregnancies. The circumstances around how they became pregnant in surrogacy were completely different.

Once pregnant, they lived in dormitories apart from their families amongst women who initially seemed like strangers, in separate, sterile worlds disconnected from their intimate lives with their husbands and children. Their routines were altered, synthetic, and removed from the context of their everyday lives. In these sequestered, women-only spaces, new routines were established wherein the mothers' bodies were carefully nurtured, iron and calcium supplements, for example, being regularly ingested so that the fetuses grew to optimal size. Their bodies were monitored through numerous blood tests and biweekly abdominal ultrasounds so that doctors could chart the growth of the babies, and the commissioning parents witness the growth of "their babies." Those nine months at the dormitory constituted an unfamiliar life event that only reinforced the reality that the impending babies did not belong to them, to be embraced in their arms, held close to their hearts, and loved through acts of caring devotion. Dorm staff and their comothers too reiterated to them that the babies they held in their wombs did not belong to them.

Whether surrogate mothers are seen as women who rent out their wombs or as wage workers, it is impossible to separate that womb or labor from that woman. Her entire being is tied to it, and in that sense, her entire self—her mind, her intellect, her emotions—is engaged in making these babies. Yet the alienness of their experiences in surrogacy marked this particular pregnancy as a period of time and experience outside their life worlds, a contractual interlude when they worked for someone else for nine months. Thus, a mother's alienation from womb, from labor, and from baby is not established *a priori*; instead, it is produced for each and every surrogate mother through the contract and through her experiences with her pregnancy.

Many surrogate mothers, in spite of that manufactured alienation, felt connected to the babies they birthed. Thirty-one-year-old Neeta, one of Kavita's friends who was waiting to become a surrogate mother, said that she would never let the surrogated baby go from her sight. It would break her heart. "After having grown the baby in my womb for so many months, how can I give her away and not feel pain," Neeta asked. She would run after the intended parents, she said, begging, pleading, and cursing if they denied her request to hold the baby. The mothers, though, were apprehensive about upsetting their recipient parents. Apparently the latter complained to Mr. Shetty if they were unhappy with their surrogate mothers. When Suma delivered her baby, for example, she had invited other residents to visit her and the baby. The intended parents were very unhappy about the crowd around their baby, and they complained. Suma was soundly reprimanded by the dorm manager, who told her, "[T]his is not a baby you have had with your husband. Why do you think you can show pride and have every one come see the baby?" Suma said she felt terrible about this.

Suma professed that the baby she surrogated looked like her second-born son. I interjected that he could not have, since the baby had no genetic connection to her or her husband. She immediately retorted with irritation in her voice, "He was in my womb, madam! For nine months. Don't you think that would have made him like one of us?" She cried often when she thought about the baby she'd given up. She said:

> Most children can only hope to provide for their parents in their old age. They hope they can earn enough and realize their duties. . . . They have that pleasure (*udhara*) of fulfilling their obligations when they grow up.[29] But this baby was able to provide for his whole family right at birth. Can you imagine his good fortune (*punya*) to have accomplished so much in his young life? . . . I tell myself this and try get some satisfaction. Otherwise it is too painful.

Suma tells herself that her surrogated baby—the baby she claimed as her fourth son—was a noble soul because he had accomplished the tasks many adult men strive hard to achieve but are unable to; though just a newborn, that baby had provided for his entire family. Suma was the one with decision-making powers in giving that baby up, but from her perspective the baby too had agency. He made a sacrifice by being apart from his mother. This supreme sacrifice on his part, of separating only so that he could provide for his brothers and parents, made him a saint in Suma's eyes. Projecting a kind of noble martyrdom onto the baby comforted Suma because she was able to justify this as his destiny, as something that was written in his stars. She was simply the conduit for a great soul to come into this world. To think otherwise, to accept the surrogated baby as just any other baby, was too painful for her.

Kavita, who has not yet been a surrogate mother, knows the process will be emotionally taxing and she "prays for strength" when it is time to give up the baby. She feels that the baby will want *her* more than she/he will want the intended parents. But Kavita says she will close her heart, focus on her own children who are dependent upon her, and give the surrogated child away. Kavita describes eloquently the emotion labors involved in giving up babies. She had to actively cast her imagination to manage her feelings, channeling her connectedness to a compulsory alienation.

Her older sister Indirani declared that "loving children is a burden" because of the responsibilities involved. In order to fulfill those maternal responsibilities to her own two children she had to suffer through degrading labor processes such as surrogacy. She could not afford any more children. Thus, even though she claimed that she had no feelings for the babies she had given up, she also explained why she *came to develop* no feelings. She repeated almost each time we met that she did not have a "sesame seed" of affection for the twin babies she had surrogated. Indirani's alienation from her pregnancy and the babies was nurtured through relentless vigilance over her emotions, lest she grew attached to those babies she had to give up.

The birth of these surrogated babies was surrounded by the violence of separation. Not only was flesh separated from flesh in that process of birth bathed in maternal blood, the babies literally being cut out of the mothers' wombs, but additionally the newborns were removed from that one presence, that of the surrogate mothers, they had known best. They went to new parents who loved them absolutely and completely from even before they were born, to be sure; but they were strangers. It is no wonder then that Suma projected nobility to the baby boy she has surrogated, and Kavita said she would pray for the strength she would need to let the baby go. The mothers felt they made huge sacrifices in order to be surrogate mothers.

Sacrifice in Labor

Value, German philosopher Georg Simmel says, "accrues to the desired object, in part or even entirely through the measure of the sacrifice demanded in acquiring it."[30] Two kinds of sacrifice, absolute and relative, are entailed in labor. Absolute sacrifice is bound up in the expenditure of labor itself because this effort is annoying and troublesome.[31] The second sort of sacrifice is the relative kind, wherein "we can attain one object only at the cost of denying ourselves another."[32] A person can choose to expend her labor on a given set of alternatives, but selecting one means other options have been relinquished. Therefore even happily performed labor is a "form of exchange entailing renunciation" and the value of objects is determined by the *sacrifice entailed in labor*.

Understanding the labor process as constituted through sacrifice is especially useful in thinking about transnational surrogacy. Bangalore's mothers point to the considerable sacrifice that their children, husbands, parents, in-laws, and real/fictive kinswomen make in order for surrogacy to be successful. The extra work that fell on kinswomen because the mothers were absent for nine months, and the renunciation of family time with loved ones were all regretted as real losses. The mothers felt their monetary compensation was inadequate because the various agents involved ignored their individual and collective efforts. But most hurtful of all was the fact that no one acknowledged their considerable efforts.

On Markets and Suffering

Yet in spite of all the sacrifices entailed, many surrogate mothers claimed that surrogacy was good employment. I was not fully convinced because their replies to my questions seemed so glib and easy. I'd approach the question differently; I'd ask them, especially if they had daughters, if they would support their daughters' decisions to pursue a similar line of employment. Almost all of them said no. But if they maintained that employment on reproductive assembly lines was good work, why did they not want their own daughters to ever sell their eggs or become surrogate mothers?

I received the hint of an answer from Indirani when I asked her whether the hormonal injections to prepare her for ova extraction and subsequently for embryo implantation were painful or scary. Was she worried about the long-term health consequences of such medical interventions? She avoided answering directly. "*Aiyo akka*," she said. "When you're poor you can't afford the luxury of thinking about discomfort." Only those who were weak or led privileged lives felt pain. And she was not privileged or weak. She was a surrogate mother because she wanted to push her family out of precarity and provide a secure economic foothold for her children. She was emphatic about not wanting the same career for her daughter. In spite of her vigorous endorsement and very active participation in Bangalore's reproductive assembly lines both as laborer and as labor recruiter, Indirani implicitly recognized the risks and degradation involved in these markets in life.

I cautioned the mothers I met about the potential negative health repercussions of repeated synthetic hormonal infusions into their bodies and repeated caesarian sections. They usually brushed aside my cautionary words. Indirani said she would worry about the long-term effects if and when they arose. There were far more pressing issues she needed to attend to at present rather than having to worry about an unforeseen future.

Pushpa, though, did not have the luxury of worrying later.[33] Of all the mothers I met, Pushpa was the only one who spoke at length of how dreadfully painful the whole process was and how she never wanted to attempt surrogacy again. Her first effort at surrogacy had resulted in an ectopic pregnancy when the implanted embryo rooted in one of her fallopian tubes. She said she was in agony a week or so after implantation, and she eventually had an excruciatingly painful miscarriage accompanied by heavy bleeding. She was in the hospital for over a week because she needed blood transfusions. Pushpa recalled that Mr. Shetty was very sympathetic during this time. He gave her approximately $600 to cover her loss of wages and follow-up gynecological visits. However, when she got better Mr. Shetty insisted that the money he had given her was a loan. He wanted her to either pay him back immediately or agree to be a surrogate mother again. Pushpa was devastated; she did not have the money to return to him, but neither did she want to put her life at risk again.

I advised her to get rid of her cell phone, change homes, and simply disappear from COTW's radar. How would her recruiting agent and Mr. Shetty track her down if she moved to a different neighborhood? The idea was not new to Pushpa; she had thought of it herself. I reassured her that she was legally entitled to half the amount she would have received for a successful surrogacy pregnancy. Mr. Shetty was deceiving her by illegally withholding money that rightfully belonged to her. And he was breaking the law by coercing her into surrogacy. That was my last meeting with Pushpa. She had taken a bus to meet me and we sat in my father's car at the Jayanagar bus stop. I called her again, but her cell phone did not work and none of the other surrogate mothers knew how to get in touch with her.

While it might seem that surrogacy is a relatively risk-free enterprise for the mothers—given that of the seventy women I met, just one of them had faced significant medical repercussions—it is more realistic to recognize that this "rate of safety" might be due to selection bias. That is, women who have medical complications have incentives to drop out and become peripheral to the networks of women moving in and out of Bangalore's reproductive industry. They are naysayers, active disbelievers, amongst a group of women who are vigorous vendors of their reproductive abilities. Women like Pushpa can testify to the risks involved, the excruciatingly painful and often humiliating processes they have endured in their failed labor attempts in Bangalore's reproductive assembly lines. They no longer sell their ova and neither are they recruiters. The real threat they pose to the system lies in their ability to dissuade others from selling their eggs and receive wages for their pregnancies. They can potentially hinder others' efforts to recruit more women into remunerative reproduction. And because of that, they are advertently and inadvertently pushed out of these networks. This was why I did not meet such individuals through the networks of surrogate mothers, ova vendors, and recruiters I'd encountered.

Pushpa was an anomaly in my study not because she suffered health consequences but because I had been able to meet her. Bangalore's reproductive industry most probably had far more casualties than its participants were willing to acknowledge. Egg retrievals and in vitro fertilizations were all relatively novel medical procedures which are not understood fully, or mastered through technological innovations. And failed pregnancies are far more frequent than most surrogacy agencies and infertility specialists in India are willing to admit.[34]

6

Fetuses as Persons, Surrogate Mothers as Nonpersons

Jeff was a gay man in his early forties living in New York, and had been in a relationship with his partner, Geoff, for over twenty years.[1] They were the fathers of two baby girls through the efforts of two Mumbai surrogate mothers who had been implanted with embryos prepared from the same egg donor, but with eggs fertilized separately by the two men's sperm. In our first telephone conversation Jeff told me, "I never in my life imagined I could get pregnant. As a gay man, and having been one for so long, I have no interest in experiencing a pregnancy. All I wanted to do was be a parent, not experience pregnancy." Yet upon receiving the news that the surrogate mothers in Mumbai had both tested positive for pregnancy, Jeff had loudly and proudly proclaimed—"*We're* pregnant!"[2]

Jocelyn, a forty-year-old straight American woman living in Chicago with her husband of ten years, after numerous failed IVF attempts was now contracting with two Delhi surrogate mothers to birth two babies. She posted on her blog, along with two images of the fetuses in the mothers' wombs: "*We* are 32 weeks pregnant and everything is going very well. We feel truly blessed and want to thank [doctors' names deleted] . . . and everyone else at [hospital's name deleted]. So here are our two gorgeous babies" (my emphasis). Along with claiming the pregnancies as belonging to her and her husband, Jocelyn thanked everyone in India except the surrogate mothers.

Not all clients express ownership over the surrogate mothers' pregnancies as do Jeff and Jocelyn. Yet enough of them do so, which warrants closer examination. In this chapter I show how intended parents cast the surrogate mothers' pregnancies as theirs, and the fetuses as fully formed persons replete with personalities, as their children. In all this, the surrogate mothers disappeared. Even as fetuses became persons, these Third World women became nonpersons. Much of the process of making and unmaking persons was facilitated by the client parents' vigorous pursuit of commodification processes. If the surrogate mothers worked hard to cultivate their alienation from the babies, the clients participated actively in commodification processes precisely because it was only through these acts that the fetus became a real and vibrant social actor. The market processes described here are in no way a castigation of the intended parents or skepticism toward the love they had for the children they had struggled so hard to bring into their lives. Instead, my purpose is to reveal that commodification and love are not antagonistic; they can indeed be complementary, with parental love abetting commodification processes, and commodification itself fostering familial emotional ties.[3]

Why Do Intended Parents Claim the Surrogate Mothers' Pregnancies as Theirs?

As progenitors, if even one person out of the couple had a genetic tie to the fetus, the clients were legally recognized parents in India. But this legal recognition depended on the client parents' countries of origin. For example, commercial surrogacy is illegal in Australia.[4] In the United States a plethora of laws regulate surrogacy; some states such as California are extremely intended-parent friendly and others such as New York do not fully recognize commercial surrogacy arrangements. Gay parents face greater challenges than straight couples because their long-term relationships may receive little or no legal recognition in their countries of origin. Their surrogacy contract can be rendered null and void if their relationship is not accorded legal recognition.[5]

Thus, clients' anxieties about their babies born in India was understandable. Because of the legal ambiguity surrounding their parental status, clients made more emphatic ownership claims to the surrogate mothers' pregnancies and the resulting babies. By doing so they established for themselves and others that the babies were truly *theirs*.

Some intended parents I spoke with recognized that the surrogate mothers *might* have greater moral claims over the babies. After all, the fetus had grown in the woman's body, literally attached to her, and was dependent on her nurturance for its growth and survival. What if the newborn and surrogate mother were closer to each other, both physically and emotionally, than the intended parents were to this newly arriving family member? Though not explicitly articulated, it became apparent when talking with intended parents that they recognized how hard it might be for surrogate mothers to give the babies away. One couple mentioned that they chose India because the surrogate mothers there had no rights over the baby they had gestated. As a result, the mothers had no legal recourse to claiming the surrogated baby, which secured the clients' parental rights to a greater degree.

For some intended parents, this anxiety over the children manifested itself over breast-feeding. Some parents and infertility doctors claimed that by not allowing surrogate mothers to breast-feed the babies they were shielding the women from the pain of separation. They gave long explanations of how hormones would flood the mothers' bodies, promoting their ties to the newborn babies they held to their breasts. Yet almost all the parents were silent about the fact that perhaps the woman might already have bonded with the baby, the surrogate mother feeling that the fetus and she existed as a single entity, living and breathing as one until the baby's birth.

One intended mother I interviewed, Elvia, was especially upset when her surrogate mother had breast-fed the newborn baby. Elvia was a forty-nine-year-old dark-skinned Latina from California who had been dealing with infertility for the past decade and had traveled to India with her husband, who was white. Through a renowned infertility specialist they contracted with an Indian surrogate mother, Mina, to have a baby for them. They used an Indian egg donor and Elvia's husband's sperm. In spite of Elvia's request that a dark-skinned egg donor be selected, her Indian doctor chose an extremely light-skinned donor and the baby was far more light-skinned than the client mother had ever imagined her child could be.[6]

Upon the baby's birth through caesarian section Mina had cried uncontrollably, and later held the baby to her breast and fed the newborn. Elvia was repulsed because the surrogate mother had not even cleaned her breast before feeding the baby. She described the mother's body as filthy and complained to the doctor, who reprimanded Mina for her unprofessional conduct. Elvia wanted to return to India to contract with Mina again, to have a second child, but this time she would take a breast pump with her so that the mother could express her milk in order to nourish the baby.

This was my first conversation with Elvia and I was troubled by it. It seems that Mina was miraculously suited to birth Elvia's baby, but she reverted to being an unfit body once he was born. Over the past two and a half years, though, I have come to appreciate this particular story differently. In subsequent conversations Elvia told me she accepted her now five-year-old son as Latino though his genetic heritage was Indian and white. What made him Latino, she wondered, other than her being a Latina mother? As a much older, dark-skinned mother with a very light-skinned child in tow, Elvia was bothered when strangers mistook her for the child's nanny. She related many incidents where people presumed she was not the mother, but a *domestica* caring for her employer's baby. This devaluation of her motherhood distressed Elvia deeply. Not only was she not the birth mother, but to make matters worse some strangers did not even acknowledge her as that child's mother.

Elvia projected the anxieties she felt onto Mina. She transferred the angst aroused in her by the social derogation of her motherhood to Mina. The net result was that both women's motherhood was negated precisely because of who they were, that is, women of color. However, unlike most other client parents Elvia had kept in touch with Mina. She now has one more child through Mina. Though it was not easy, Elvia explained that she wanted to honor the woman who gave birth to her children. She felt morally obligated to continue that fraught relationship both for Mina's and the children's sake.

Given the morally competing claims on the baby that arose in transnational surrogacy, and the social misrecognition and subsequent denial of parentage to women of color and gay fathers, the intended parents' anxious desire to establish "ownership" over the fetuses was understandable. They claimed the surrogate's pregnancy as their own, declaring themselves to be pregnant, imaginatively reassigning the surrogate mother's labor to their own bodies. In this process of transference the material reality of the surrogate mother disappeared, and all that mattered was the familial dyad composed of the growing fetuses and the intended parents. The surrogate mothers, never in a social relationship with the intended parents to begin with, faded from existence. In all this, the opposite happened to the fetus.

Fetuses as Real Social Actors

Still a future being whose existence depended wholly upon the surrogate mother, the fetus materialized as a person just weeks into the pregnancy. A large part of why the intended parents attributed such solidity to the fetus was precisely because it was still immaterial; that is, it had not yet manifested itself as a full human. But its potential to be one animated the intended parents, who imagined it already as a real child who would enrich their lives. In order to connect with the eventual child and to prepare for the arrival of one or more babies into their lives, clients spoke of the pregnancy as their own and flooded their blogs with ultrasound images and countdowns to delivery dates.

One strand of feminist literature on motherhood discusses how the fuzzy fetal ultrasound images are imagined as full-term babies, with many to-be-mothers collecting and sharing fetal images with friends and family.[7] Client parents who worked with Indian surrogate mothers were no different. Their blogs and the fetal images on their social media were affirmations of parental lineage, with the assemblage of online images of nurseries, strollers, baby clothes, and ultrasounds as self-representations of family. Almost all the intended parents I interviewed uploaded pictures of the fetuses on their blogs and social media, lovingly and with great humor, attributing all sorts of characteristics to them.

Carey and Drew, Jewish fathers living in Atlanta, said that they did not want to speak of the baby before she arrived because they did not want to bring the evil eye upon their family. Yet even they could not resist posting pictures of the fetus on their blogs. Another gay father (not interviewed) wrote in his blog, "I just wanna pinch those little chubby cheeks!!! I think that's his/her little hand in front of his/her mouth. But, I can't help but imagine that he/she is singing a happy tune or whistling the time away. (Now that I look again, maybe it looks like he/she is spitting!)." Quinn and Antonio, a gay Texan couple, facetiously wrote in their blog that one of their twins "looked a bit evil, as if rubbing palms together planning world domination."

In addition to making the blurred, indistinct images in the ultrasounds into real people with personalities, the intended parents began nesting. They converted their homes to make space for their babies, anticipating their needs, and imagining what the children might need or enjoy. They moved into larger houses or closer to their natal families. They prepared elaborate nurseries by painting walls, buying furniture, and hanging pictures. They bought strollers, car seats, clothing, and bottles. In this process of buying the accouterments necessary for their baby, they marked for themselves how their lives and their relationship with the world around them would change forever. These nesting activities were accompanied by baby showers, which were rituals that affirmed to society at large that the intended parents and the babies were a family unit even before the arrival of the baby.

In so-called normal pregnancies too, individuals engage in conversations about the baby prior to its arrival, replete with baby showers that anthropologists identify as "consumer rites of American culture."[8] For most Americans the entire pregnancy is marked by ritualistic consumptive acts. Patterns of consumption change; that is, to-be-parents buy car seats, organic foods, and such. But more important, the meaning of consumption itself changes. For to-be-parents, especially expectant mothers, consumption becomes "invested with new levels of moral significance—consumption is cast as an act of maternal love, and an expression of a woman's character and powers of self-discipline, even as consumption is also seen to literally create the fetal body."[9]

These acts of consumption were very significant for the intended parents because the surrogate mother's pregnancy and the growing fetus were unfamiliar; they were events occurring halfway across the world to women with whom they had no connection. Because of language, class, and other cultural barriers the intended parents were unable to correspond with their surrogate mothers. All they received over email, if they were lucky enough to work with doctors who cared, were biweekly ultrasound images of fetal growth. And perhaps a photograph of the smiling surrogate mother with her distended belly growing "their baby." The doctors tried to facilitate the intended parents' closeness to the fetuses through regular email updates about fetal growth in order to make it more of a solid presence for their clients.

The clients actively cast their imaginations and emotions to make the fetus a full person in their lives in order to cement their relationship with the forthcoming baby. Contrary to the surrogate mothers who were physically, emotionally and intellectually engaged with that fetus, and who worked hard to create pregnancy as an alienable wage labor process and the baby as a commodity, the intended parents, who were in no way physically connected with the fetus, did the opposite; they worked hard emotionally and intellectually to create connections to the "baby." Much of this bonding was created through consumerism, acts of acquiring objects that signified the arrival of the baby and their own impending parenthood.

The bonds they felt with the as-yet-unborn babies were especially palpable in the poignant stories they shared about the surrogate mothers' pregnancy losses or the death of newborns. Bruce and Will's first attempt at surrogacy in Delhi was one such story. The surrogate mother had a difficult pregnancy and went into labor prematurely. One baby boy was stillborn, and the other baby, Ben, was in neonatal care for five weeks. The fathers kept an agonizing vigil by their son's bedside for weeks as he struggled to pull through before deciding to take him off life support at the recommendation of doctors when his condition deteriorated irreversibly. They presently have two daughters through two Delhi surrogate mothers, but the loss of their twin sons has stayed with them.

For many of the intended parents, the fetuses began to develop into persons early in the surrogate mother's pregnancy. This bonding was especially apparent when they talked about how deeply conflicted they felt over the selective reduction, or abortion, of fetuses. Many intended parents said that the doctors they worked with had implanted up to four embryos in the surrogate mothers' wombs. In some cases, when they worked with two surrogate mothers, each woman was implanted with four fetuses to increase the chances of a successful delivery. The intended parents were faced with the possible scenario of taking eight babies home. In these situations doctors selectively reduced the fetuses, that is, they aborted them until an ideal number was reached for the sake of the surrogate mother, fetal health, and often, at the clients' requests. At these times client parents were heartbroken.

James and Scott, who lived in Melbourne, Australia, experienced such a situation when all four embryos implanted in the surrogate mother started to grow into fetuses. The doctor got in touch with the men to explain she had to reduce two fetuses. They were inconsolable because abortion went against their beliefs and they mourned what they said felt like the death of their two babies. If selective reduction goes against their religious beliefs or ethics, then why do clients ask for two surrogate mothers, with each woman implanted with four embryos? One could imagine that they anticipated fetal reduction, but that was not necessarily the case.

For straight couples, given their long histories of infertility and struggles with attempting to get pregnant, and for gay men who had been discriminated against in the adoption market, the very notion of having children seemed remote. One straight intended mother, an American, wrote in her blog about the two fetuses growing in two surrogate mothers' bodies in Delhi:

> The last few weeks I have been trying to work out how to phrase things regarding the babies. Every time I talk about them, or a future with them,

> it's like I have to include little lines such as 'if it happens'–'if it works out this time'-'hopefully if . . .' It is kind of tiring, but after such major disappointments, I find it so hard to chat in a fully positive tone. Hopefully one day soon . . .

I have not interviewed this woman who had undergone numerous infertility cycles, a failed cycle with an Indian surrogate mother, and the loss of twins at twenty-two weeks' gestational age through another surrogate mother in India. I reproduce her words from her blog because it best exemplifies many intended parents' feelings that a baby may never happen. Thus, when Indian infertility doctors recommended that they contract with two surrogate mothers and implant four embryos each in both women, the intended parents often did not process the fact that the doctors might have to "selectively reduce" the fetuses. All they wanted was babies to nurture and the fact that they might have "multiples," in the face of their immense losses, seemed impossible. And so, when eventually faced with the scenario of fetal reduction, they were devastated.

Quinn and Antonio in Houston had a much more complex take on selective reduction than most other interviewees. They wrote in their blog that they hoped the procedure was not too painful or frightening for "the sweet, cheerful-looking woman" who was carrying their children. They believed that it was a woman's right to choose what she did with her body, and if she wanted to carry twins instead of quadruplets, then it was her choice. After all, wasn't "choosing to become a surrogate mother another expression of that freedom?" Being pregnant with quadruplets, they recognized, increased the health risks both for the surrogate mother and the babies. Moreover, they had the financial resources to raise only two children, not four. They claimed it was too early for them to feel too strongly about the fetuses, and though selective reduction was their only choice, Quinn couldn't help thinking that this would profoundly affect the rest of their lives. He was not sure why the two eliminated embryos were chosen. And he kept thinking, "[I]f that nearly random needle had chosen another, who would they have become? What was lost? And what will we tell our kids if they ever ask 'what, you mean it could have been me?'" He later added that the most important thing he'd tell his two children was that he and Antonio "got exactly the kids we were meant to have." Quinn and Antonio expressed ambivalence; they spoke of the mother's potential anxiety regarding selective reduction, yet they also spoke of their very real needs as a family. They indicated that the fetuses were not people, yet they acknowledged that selective reduction had very real consequences. Perhaps randomly, they had been assigned their children.

All this emotional labor, essential to building a bond with the fetus even before it had become a full, independent individual being, succeeded for the intended parents. By imagining the pregnancy as theirs, creatively casting how the future baby might be, and making space for the little ones in their lives, the intended parents created bonds with the fetuses that felt very real to them even before they went to pick up those babies. They spoke of loving the babies even before they had arrived into this world. While such a love might seem inauthentic because they had conjured her into being, loving her as a concept rather than building their love on a real knowledge of her, such love was also essential to preparing themselves emotionally for the arrival of the babies. By imagining not-as-yet-real people as real individuals, and by mentally erasing the surrogate mother because her pregnancy was really theirs and the resulting baby was theirs in every sense, the intended parents established themselves as the authentic parents. In the process, however, the surrogate mother who had made the baby evaporated from their lives, and from existence.

Ephemeral Mothers

Steve and Stephanie, a white couple in their mid-thirties, lived in Boston. Stephanie knew she was unable to have children when she met Steve and they began researching their options to grow their family almost immediately upon getting married. With her eggs and his sperm to prepare embryos, all they needed was a surrogate mother to carry the fetus to term. They did not have the funds to pursue domestic surrogacy; when Steve suggested that they go to Delhi, Stephanie demurred. She felt that she could not relate to the surrogate mother and comprehend what it felt like for the other woman to be pregnant with her baby. Finally she relented when faced with the costs of a domestic surrogacy. Thus, for some clients it was not just the baby that they sought but also access to the *experience* of pregnancy by having the surrogate mother elucidate what her body was going through, and what it felt like to have the fetus growing within her.[10]

However, surrogacy in India did not afford intended parents vicarious access to pregnancy experiences because of language barriers, but more important, because of the institutional barriers enforced by the surrogacy agencies. Some parents explained that they went to considerable lengths but were unable to develop any meaningful communications with surrogate mothers because recruiting agents, doctors, and other hospital staff interceded between the two parties. Bruce and Will, a gay couple in their late thirties living close to Perth, Australia, explained further. They had met their two surrogate mothers for the first time at the delivery of their two girl babies, and then the second time ten days after birth. It was not the men's choice, but the infertility doctors stipulated that the surrogate mothers not breast-feed the babies, hold them, or even be near them. When the surrogate mothers met the fathers and the babies, each woman held the child she had birthed for the first time ever. Bruce prepared five sentences in Hindi to read to the mothers to express his gratitude for the gift of fatherhood they had bestowed on them. The translator translated their questions about how the pregnancy went, what it was like, and how they felt, but Bruce and Will emphasized that in spite of their best efforts, communication was hard. The infertility doctor and hospital staff intervened in ways that made authentic interaction impossible. The fathers wanted to send the surrogate mothers photos of the girls every year so they could see how they grew, but the surrogacy agency and the infertility doctors forbade them to correspond with the mothers directly. They had to send the pictures to the agency that had facilitated the surrogacy, and the staff there would forward them to the mothers. Bruce and Will hoped the surrogate mothers received these regular updates, but they had no way of knowing for sure.

Others, however, had no interest in having any connection with the surrogate mothers. I asked Jeff if he had conversed with the two surrogate mothers who had borne Geoff's and his babies during or after their pregnancies, and he replied: "I never in my life imagined I could get pregnant. As a gay man, and having been one for so long, I have no interest in experiencing a pregnancy. All I wanted to do was be a parent, not experience pregnancy." That, he noted, was something that heterosexual couples—specifically intended mothers—felt and wanted, and not gay couples. He explained that straight women tried hard to converse with and relate to the surrogate mother in order to comprehend what pregnancy might feel like.

Not all straight women met the standards of Jeff's stereotypical client mother. One intended mother whom I have not interviewed, who had twin babies in Anand, Gujarat, explained on her blog:

> In comparing Indian surrogacy with surrogacy in the U.S., I was attracted to the forced distance in our relationship. In the U.S., I could imagine hanging out with my surrogate on a Friday night, watching movies and eating root beer floats. We'd be besties . . . but then she'd deliver my baby (or babies) and what? Would we stay friends? Would we vacation together? Would my kids know her as surri? Would she feel a "special connection" with my kid? Did I want that? It could get awkward, fast. Kailash and I don't speak the same language. She wanted to hold the babies and we let her. We took a bunch of photos together and will give her some prints before we leave. We smile and try to communicate, taking advantage of a translator whenever we find one. We really have tried to treat her well and with respect, but we aren't best friends. I don't have her cellphone number and if I try to send pictures of C and O as they get older, I've heard they won't realistically get to her.

Pedro Paulo, a single, upper-middle-class gay father in his late forties, and a recent immigrant to the United States from Brazil, had a more complicated story of why he preferred the enforced anonymity of surrogacy in India. Pedro Paulo had first attempted to have a child through domestic surrogacy. He said that the domestic surrogacy agency claimed that the entire arrangement would cost him approximately $70,000, but new charges kept coming up and he was constantly being billed for this or that procedure. By the end of the entire process he had spent close to $100,000 which, he took pains to explain, was not necessarily egregious; but what bothered him was that in spite of all the money spent, he was not able to have a child. The surrogate mother attempted one pregnancy and miscarried. Pedro Paulo was emotionally devastated. To make matters worse, he had developed a caring relationship with the surrogate mother who was from a small town in the Midwest. In spite of their class and cultural differences, he said, he considered her his friend. He said it was very weird because he did not want to pursue a second round of embryo implantation with her, but he felt compelled to do so because of their relationship. The second time too the implantation failed. When he terminated his contract with her it felt like a breakup.

"Here I am, a gay man, breaking up with a straight woman," he said with laughter in his voice. The surrogate mother was eager to try again the third time around and attempted to coax him, but his heart was not in it. He wondered whether she wanted to attempt another pregnancy in order to help him out because of their friendship, or, whether the loss of money was the motivating factor. In the end, he said, it was both; she genuinely wanted him to have a child, and she genuinely wanted that money. Pedro Paulo explained that terminating his contract with the American woman felt not just like the death of his dream, but it was also the end of an intense relationship with her. He found the entire process deeply painful, especially because they had nothing in common other than the potential baby, and once that potential disappeared, there was nothing to sustain their friendship.

He was much happier when he contracted with an Indian surrogate mother in Delhi. He had two failures there too, but they did not feel as devastating as the ones in the United States. Right when he had given up all hope, the surrogate mother in Delhi contracted on his behalf got pregnant and carried the baby to term. After five surrogacy attempts, two in the United States and three in India, Pedro Paulo now has a one-year-old son. Overall, he felt far better about pursuing surrogacy in India than in the United States not because it was cheaper, but because he was shielded from the emotional highs and lows, and from forming caring ties with the surrogate mother. The businesslike transactions, facilitated by the vast differences in class, culture, and geographical location, protected him from forming any bonds with the surrogate mother. He could guard himself from being emotionally affected when the Indian mothers miscarried, and he could walk away with the baby once she gave birth, Pedro Paulo and his son in a familial dyad. She had to necessarily disappear as a person in order for the entire process to be less fraught for him.

Like Pedro Paulo, Jeff maintained that working with Indian surrogate mothers minimized their interactions, and therefore made the whole process emotionally easier for him and his partner. Jeff felt absolved from being present, from having to express his excitement about every aspect of the pregnancy and to otherwise communicate appropriate emotions at the appropriate times. He found it far easier to deal with the whole exchange as a solely contractual one, with his emotions kept to a bare minimum. I was initially appalled at what amounted to Jeff's callousness, but over subsequent conversations I grew to understand that his and Geoff's relationship with the two surrogate mothers was emotionally fraught for the two men. Jeff told me that he had been with his partner for eighteen years when they decided upon surrogacy in India. They had earlier attempted domestic open adoption prior to this decision, and had even been selected as recipients by a birth mother. But the mother—with whom they had developed a close friendship—changed her mind upon the birth of her child. Jeff acknowledged that she had every right to change her mind, and he even supported her decision to keep her baby. But the whole process had been an emotional roller coaster for him. He did not want any ties with birth mothers, surrogate or otherwise, again. Maintaining a strictly contractual relationship with the surrogate mothers, where they received money for the babies they had birthed, was the best way by which Jeff could protect himself.

I asked Jeff in an email exchange if he and Geoff were supported in their parenting efforts. Together with various parents who had used the services of Indian surrogate mothers like them, Jeff mentioned the nurse and chauffeur who had assisted them in Mumbai:

> Usha and Parmesh are very dear to me as they were instrumental in helping us navigate a completely foreign country and getting our children home. Above and beyond their professional services, being a month in India, I got to know them well personally. I still call Dalia my little *Gudia Rani* and Sarah my little *Sona Rani* courtesy of Usha. . . . I'm probably spelling those incorrectly. I just wish I had the resources to bring them stateside as they have both expressed interest in leaving India.[11]

Though Jeff distanced himself and his family from the surrogate mothers, he felt deeply indebted to the babies' Indian nurse Usha who assisted them during their month long stay in Mumbai. And he was grateful to Parmesh who chauffeured them in Mumbai. He still called his daughters, now three-year-old toddlers, by the nicknames Usha had given them. If he had had the means, Jeff indicated he would sponsor their travel to the United States so that they could be a part of his, Geoff's, and their daughters' lives.

This email exchange with Jeff illustrates what many intended parents felt; they did not avoid relationships with all Indian caregivers but only with their surrogate mothers, who seemed to arouse anxiety in them. The question then arises, Why did the mothers, by their very presence, cause discomfort in the intended parents?

Though none of the intended parents admitted it outright, some of them seemed to recognize that the process of getting pregnant, of being separated from their own families and young children, and of giving up the baby must have been very difficult for the surrogate mothers. Moreover, as I discuss in the next chapter, some felt a profound sense of debt to the mothers but were unable to adequately express their gratitude. They recognized that the immensity of the sacrifice made by the surrogate mothers was more than the sacrifices made by other kinds of workers in the labor market; that producing another human being was not the same as producing a chair or car, for example. More was involved. As pregnant women, the surrogate mothers had no control over the life that grew in them, which seemed to have a volition of its own. Regardless of whether they felt like they were actively engaged, whether they slept, overate, or missed a meal, much like a bee that instinctively makes a hive or a spider that spins its web, the mothers' bodies spontaneously nurtured and grew that fetus. And much like that architect that Marx describes, they knew that the "product" their bodies had made, the baby they gave birth to, would accumulate a history of her own. However, the organization of market exchange negated the mothers' total emotional, intellectual, and physical immersion in producing the babies. Some intended parents recognized that they too were complicit in invalidating the mothers' considerable efforts.

Some parents' feelings of indebtedness were complicated by the fact that they felt that perhaps the newborn babies were closer to the mothers than to them. They were justifiably reluctant to bring in another person, especially the woman who had given birth to "their" child, into their lives. What moral rights would this woman have over the child? What rights would they have in denying the surrogate mother access to the baby she had birthed? And might the newborn respond more strongly to her than to them? These were very real fears for the new parents, but they could shield themselves from their fears through the exchange of money for the pregnancy and baby. Upon paying money, they were able to exit with what they so desperately wanted. The transfer of money to the surrogate mother signaled her erasure from their lives.[12]

Much as consumers often do not reflect on the labor that goes into making the products they consume in commodity production, the parents too did not ruminate on the surrogate mother's labor. Or if they did, they maintained that she had willingly cut all her ties to the baby upon surrendering it. Engaging in market relations, then, allowed the clients to eliminate the producer. By eliminating her, they recast her labor effort in pregnancy as theirs. And they asserted that they were the baby's true and only parents because this baby existed through their intentions. Through their intentions they had engaged in the market for surrogacy, which had ultimately resulted in this baby. They, then, were the true creators of the baby. In claiming the infants as theirs the intended parents obliterated the surrogate mother's reproductive labor and mythologized the babies' origins.[13]

The surrogate mothers had no choice in the matter. In Bangalore they could not meet their "recipient" parents until the fourth month of their pregnancy. If they miscarried before then, they had no clue for whom they were pregnant and on whose account they had suffered. Surrogate mother Indirani believed this was better for the clients; she maintained that because success rates are low, when mothers miscarried clients were not as devastated as they would be if they were involved in the pregnancy right from the embryo transfer. But was she not curious about her recipients? I asked her. She laughed and said that yes she was, but she was poor and did not have the luxury of demanding to meet the recipients. And she had no say in maintaining or ending any relationship with them once they left her world with their babies in their arms.

7

Surrogacy as a Gift

So far I have discussed how surrogate mothers and client parents held onto surrogacy as a market exchange. This chapter, instead, maps how the various agents involved cast surrogacy as a gift exchange. Adrienne Arieff, a thirty-six-year-old marketing specialist in San Francisco and author of a book on surrogacy, says that when she first met her Gujarati surrogate mother, Vaina, who birthed twins for her, Arieff wanted them to operate as social equals engaging in a business transaction. But when she returned for the delivery of the twins, the business relationship transitioned into something more. She elaborates:

> We'd do things like braid each other's hair, do each other's makeup. We don't speak the same language so the relationship was based on these basic human principles and exchanges. We'd take short walks, watch movies, some Indian films. I got this drum set, and we played that a couple of times. Music, we really bonded on music and had fun making fools of ourselves. There were lots of iPhone films and looking at films together and sitting around doing nothing. We'd look at magazines I'd brought. I think her favorite was when I bought Toblerone chocolate.[1]

Arieff says of her experience with surrogacy: "There, in the 107 degree heat of Indian summer, I discovered that parenthood was possible, but it would require *a gift from a perfect stranger* . . . . What she did for me is the most generous act I could have ever imagined."[2] Arieff now travels to Gujarat once a year to visit Vaina and update her on the twin girls. Though we never hear about the relationship through Vaina's perspective, the marketing specialist is happy to see that the surrogate mother's life has improved.

Most client parents I interviewed did not cast surrogacy as a gift. But two individuals who did so repeatedly were Ed and Martin, two gay fathers in their mid-forties. They were raising three daughters in Dallas born through two surrogate mothers in Delhi. Writing about the ambivalence involved in any kind of intimate labor, especially in caring for children, Ed said that their *au pair* who helped with their three daughters had "become an important part of our family well beyond caretaker of our girls. . . . [She] will be sorely missed when her tenure is over." He expected the separation would be "painful to her as well, having spent a few years helping our girls find their way in their toddler world" (email exchange, April 20, 2012). But she had a choice, he said; she could continue to be a part of their worlds. The surrogate mothers who worked with Ed and Martin, however, did not have that choice. In spite of their efforts the men were unable to keep in touch with the women because there was "a curtain of certain secrecy" that was controlled by their clinic, and "complicated by language, geography, and poor understanding of the ultimate motivation of the surrogate's goals/needs." Clients had to trust their doctors and intermediary agents who insisted on the anonymous nature of the transaction (pers. comm. over email, March 21, 2012).

Ed described the uncertainty he and Martin felt about this enforced anonymity:

> I do understand the need for anonymity in the surrogacy process in India . . . and I think most people that travel this path convince themselves that the surrogates have found a way to cope with whatever detachment or pain they may encounter because "it's the way it is. . . ." We certainly did. We were told it was fine and fulfilled all the parts of the deal that we intended, paid our bill, and returned home. But, the more I think about it, the more I feel it's set up that way to be convenient for intended parents to neatly wrap up any perceived emotion that the surrogate may have in order to preserve the business of the transaction.

In a subsequent email Ed ironically paraphrased Brecht, noting, "The powerful of the earth can create poverty . . . we just can't bear to look at it" (pers. comm., May 22, 2012). He wanted intended parents to take greater responsibility toward the surrogate mothers because it would be better for all to maintain some connection beyond pregnancy and childbirth. Ed continued:

> I wish for our beloved surrogates that they would know—with unquestionable certainty—that they have changed every single aspect of our lives, giving us colors and emotion we didn't know existed. We give them all of that credit. Without them, we'd just be a couple of gay guys who live a privileged life. It makes me sad to think they may not know that. Or ever have to question the greatness of their gift in a dark hour where they feel pain or regret about their choice to have completed a pregnancy for someone else. I don't know if other parents feel the same way—I suspect some do and some allow the convenience of the process to check a box and move on with life.

He said that they had "an unpaid debt of enormous gratitude" that they needed to make good on; he hoped to get that opportunity soon. Both the surrogate mothers' names were in their "church program, remembered in prayer for months before and after" the three girls were born. He claimed, "[T]here isn't a day that passes that I don't think about both of them, even briefly, as I go about the incredible tasks of raising three girls" (pers. comm., March 21, 2012). Their efforts paid off two years later, in 2014, when Martin traveled to India with gifts for the two women and their families, and with news and photographs of the girls. The fathers in Dallas were committed to building on this reunion and developing a relationship with the mothers in Delhi.

The one other person who tried to keep up a relationship with her surrogate mother was Elvia. Though fraught and difficult, she worked hard to stay in touch with Mina who birthed her two children for her.

She said she was committed to this relationship because of her own sense of ethics and morality, and felt it was the right thing to do for Mina, and for all the children involved. Unlike Ed, Martin, and Elvia, however, most client parents professed that if the surrogate mothers had given them babies then they had given the mothers a large sum of money that transformed the lives of the women and their families. The gift exchange, in their perspective, was equal.

Money for Babies as a Mutually Beneficial Exchange

Most intended parents, to use Ed's words, "checked a box and moved on with life," holding onto the belief that their money for babies was an equitable and just exchange. Surrogacy agencies and infertility doctors too insisted that money for babies was a fair and equal exchange. For example, Dr. Nayna Patel of Anand, Gujarat, who is arguably the best known provider of surrogacy in India, claims:

> There is this one woman who desperately needs a baby and cannot have her own child without the help of a surrogate. And at the other end there is this woman who badly wants to help her family. . . . If this female wants to help the other one why not allow that? It's not for any bad cause. They're helping one another to have a new life in this world.[3]

Her client, author Adrienne Arieff who believes that surrogacy is a gift, also says that she wanted her money to help a poor mother there. She notes:

> [A] woman going through the risks of labor for another family clearly deserves to be paid. To me, this was not exploitation. This was a win-win, allowing the surrogate to have a brighter future and the couple to have a child. If my money was going to benefit an Indian woman financially for a service she willingly provided, I preferred that it be a poor woman who really needed help because the money that a surrogate earns in India is, to be blunt, life-changing.[4]

Client parents said that the one persistent criticism they faced in their decision to pursue transnational surrogacy was that they were wealthy Westerners who took advantage of oppressed and easily exploitable Third World women. In response the commissioning parents pointed to the discrimination they faced when attempting to adopt; and they pointed to the social isolation they felt in being childless. They maintained that transnational surrogacy was a life-altering experience for them *and* for the surrogate mothers who ostensibly transitioned out of poverty. For example, Phil and Colin, a white gay Midwestern couple in their early forties, believed that their pursuit of surrogacy in Delhi helped enable their two surrogate mothers to make ends meet. To those who criticized them Phil posed the question, "What have you ever done to make the lives of these women better? You're so quick to judge me, but I have. I can point to two people who have homes and have sent their kids to school as a result of our direct involvement with them." In this manner many client parents cast their market pursuit of parenthood as a form of altruism which transformed surrogate mothers' lives.

Amrita Pande (2011) sees a similar pattern of expressed beneficence by the American client mothers she interviewed. She notes that these sorts of narratives are similar to the rescue narratives conveyed by parents who engage in transnational adoption that represent children from the global South as "waiting children" who have been saved by loving Western parents. These rescue fantasies posit parents as inherently benevolent actors who save a child, while simultaneously eliding the socioeconomic conditions that led the biological parents to relinquish that child in the first place. Even though there was no ostensibly abandoned child that needed rescuing in surrogacy, the intended mothers Amrita Pande interviewed truly believed they were on missions of compassion because they had liberated one impoverished Indian woman and her children from the clutches of poverty.[5] Their global pursuit of parenthood made them supreme moral actors who contributed to building families in the West and the East. They might act like rational market actors, but they were socially responsible individuals who put their money to a good cause because they provided employment to Third World women, and thereby benefited Third World children.

However, contrary to what surrogacy agencies, infertility doctors, and some intended parents declared, commercial surrogacy was not a "win-win" exchange where both parties received equal rewards. Instead, the intended parents gained considerably more, but they had nothing in their possession that could fundamentally alter the surrogate mothers' worlds in contrast to what the mothers had given them. Hence, it was perhaps not surprising that they cast their monetary contributions to the surrogate mothers' lives as larger than warranted. They sincerely believed that the money they gave in return for their babies was just as life changing for the mothers as the babies were for them. To openly acknowledge otherwise was perhaps deeply shaming because they might have felt like they were making use of another person's economic precarity. However, they were not alone in casting their market pursuits as charitable acts.

There are many firms in India like Creative Options Trust for Women (COTW). They are registered as not-for-profit social work organizations because they claim their economic pursuits are charitable. The notion that surrogacy agencies double as social work organizations is endorsed by India's Assisted Reproductive Technologies (ART) Bill of 2010, which encourages third party agencies, that is, surrogacy agencies to act independently of infertility doctors ostensibly to protect the best interests of the surrogate mother. Dr. R. S. Sharma, Deputy Director General of the Indian Council for Medical Research, and member-secretary of the ART Bill's drafting committee, says the reason for barring infertility specialists from hiring women directly is to "create a safe distance between the clinic and the surrogate to avoid unethical practices. . . . IVF [in vitro fertilization] clinics should only be concerning themselves with science."[6]

The framing of businesses such as surrogacy as social work endeavors has a much larger context. Many market activities that focus on Third World indigent women are perceived as socially responsible endeavors and not simply as money-making enterprises. That is, they are forms of social entrepreneurism. The most famous exponent of the idea of social entrepreneurism is Dr. Muhammad Yunus, founder of the microcredit Grameen Bank for women and winner of the 2006 Nobel Peace Prize. Dr. Yunus argues that entrepreneurs, which by his definition would include founders of surrogacy agencies, are driven by two motivations "which are mutually exclusive, but equally compelling—a) maximization of profit and b) doing good to people and the world." In this frame, profit making and humanitarian efforts are not at odds with each other but are mutually constitutive. He trusts that all the world's social problems can be addressed through "social businesses"—be it health care, financial services, information technology, and renewable energy for the poor. He believes that his Grameen Bank, that provided microcredit for rural Bangladeshi women, inculcated them into market behavior, which subsequently empowered them by teaching them responsibility and helping them develop self-respect.[7]

Surrogacy agencies and some infertility doctors in India made strikingly similar arguments. That is, being paid for pregnancy empowered working-class Indian women. They had previously birthed children for free, but now they were able to develop self-confidence and self-worth because they were being paid for it and had control over a good sum of money. The late Dr. Sulochana Gunasheela, the leading Bangalore infertility specialist, believed that commercial, gestational surrogacy empowered working-class women with greater self-confidence and social power.[8] In her extensive experience as an infertility specialist since the late 1980s she said she had come to learn that altruistic surrogacy in India tended to be exploitative. Upper-middle-class families felt entitled to poorer women's bodies and labor, and the surrogate mothers were unable to avoid the demands placed on their reproductive abilities, especially if their families had a long history of dependent interactions with their employers or wealthier relatives. Many clients assumed that they had already assisted poorer relatives or working-class women by paying for the latter's children's tuition or giving the women or their husbands employment. Commercial, gestational surrogacy, according to Dr. Gunasheela, circumvented such exploitative relations because the surrogate mother could now receive a salary for her work in producing that baby. Unfettered by social relations of commitment and compulsion to the commissioning family, she could use the money she earned to potentially negotiate a powerful position for herself within her own nuclear and extended household. Dr. Gunasheela believed women workers could be empowered by marketing their pregnancies.

My intention here is not to claim that infertility doctors and intended parents were deliberately lying to their critics, acting in bad faith, or fooling themselves into believing that they made a difference in the mothers' lives. The money they gave to the surrogate mothers *could* potentially make a difference; for example, Adrienne Arieff believes that the money she gave to Vaina for bearing twins "was the equivalent of 10 to 15 years of salary."[9] This may certainly have been the case for Vaina, but for the women I met in Bangalore, because they had already incurred expenses in preparing for surrogacy, their take-home pay was less than $4,000, which turned out to be far less than they had imagined. Their earnings amounted to approximately two years of salary; wages for surrogacy, to be blunt, was not life-changing for a majority of the surrogate mothers I met. The women's earnings from selling their eggs or surrogacy dissipated rapidly.

The various agents involved in surrogacy, right from the doctors to the agents who ran the surrogacy agencies, blamed the mothers for dissipating their surrogacy wages. For example, Dr. Nayna Patel helped the mothers manage their money because "we will not know what they are going to do with such a big amount of money." If they wanted to buy a piece of land or otherwise invest their money, Dr. Patel is quoted as saying, "we get them the best deal."[10] The mothers too believed themselves to be gullible fools, bad managers of money, and uneducated dupes with not enough common sense to save their money or make wise investments. The Bangalore mothers contemptuously described themselves or others who had not pulled themselves out of poverty as women who did not have even three cents' worth of substance in her head.[11] Thus they faulted themselves; in spite of being "given the opportunity" to pull themselves up by their uteri, if you will, they were unable to do so.

Bangalore, however, was an expensive city. Working-class families paid up to $2,000 as security deposit and monthly rents of up to $50 for small, one- to two-room homes with potable water facilities in the kitchen and a bathroom they shared with six to eight neighbors. Food was expensive, as were utilities. Monthly cell phone charges needed to be budgeted in. The children's tuition cost money. In-laws and parents often fell sick and some of their husbands were alcoholics who did not have steady employment. Yet other husbands were either skilled workers in the construction business or they were auto drivers, but their livelihoods were severely affected by recessions that depressed the construction industry and changed transportation patterns in the city.[12] And employment in the garment industry for women, so intimately tied to the global market, was volatile. The women's families were either flush with money or had none at all. The only stable factor in their lives was their economic instability. Consequently many families took on substantial loans to tide over the weeks or months of underemployment or joblessness.

I grew to realize that the value of money differed from person to person, depending on their circumstances or more specifically, on their class status. Four thousand U.S. dollars might stretch much further for a middle-class person with economic means than it could for a working-class person. The former could invest it, use it for a vacation, buy a luxury item, or make a partial down payment toward a house. Middle-class people tend not to have such pressing needs for which the money is required. They also tend not to have extended family members who need cash immediately in order to get them out of financial crises. If they do, they can turn to banks that potentially deem them low-risk bets because of their net worth. Or these needy family members can depend on a larger network of magnanimous relatives who can loan them relatively small amounts of cash as short-term interest-free loans.

When they received that $4,000 in their hands, the surrogate mothers were almost always the only individual in their extended families to have held that much liquid capital. As a result, other family members who needed assistance petitioned the women to direct some money their way. The surrogate mothers and their husbands had debts that needed to be serviced, deposits to make toward renting livable homes, private education for their children to be paid for, sick relatives who needed immediate attention, or small agricultural holdings that needed capital until the next big drought wiped out all their prior investments. The surrogate mothers and their extended families lived in financially precarious states with no safety net. They were constantly short of money in their struggle to make a decent life. Any cash inflow immediately flowed out. Although they endeavored to create some sense of financial security, that security eluded them repeatedly. So they actively recruited others into reproductive assembly lines, and simultaneously wanted to become surrogate mothers all over again so that they might wrest a little more value out of their bodies while they still had youth and robust fertility on their side.

There were some client parents who believed that this desperation made the surrogate mothers dangerous social agents capable of wreaking havoc over their orderly lives. I describe in the following section someone from that thin slice of the consumer market—I have just one example—who professed that he wanted nothing more to do with surrogate mothers, those ostensibly depraved individuals, once he took "his" babies back.

Degrading Work and Degraded Workers

When I first began research on surrogacy I read a series of blogs maintained by intended parents and I wrote to them asking to talk with them about their experiences regarding surrogacy in India. Most of them ignored my request, and some complied. The only confrontational interaction I had was with an intended father who signed his email "John." In reply to my email soliciting an interview, he wrote back:

> I'm very skeptical in participating in something like this because the truth be told most coverage of the international surrogacy practice tends to be very negative: rich Westerners exploiting poor, down-trodden Third Worlders is usually the gist of most articles or video clips I have seen. Which actually is as far from the truth as it gets. The women (and their husbands) who participate in this trade, be they in India or elsewhere, are as entrepreneurial as they get. They are in this for the money and could care less about anything else. I can relay horror stories about how IPs [intended parents] have been burned but don't have the time for that. The fact that you are making a distinction between "transnational" surrogacy and domestic surrogacy performed here in the US, which has been happening for decades, leads me to believe that perhaps there is a political agenda here. I am not interested in being a part of that.

I reproduce this email text *not* to point out the suspicions John had regarding my research. Instead, my reason for doing so is to highlight the suspicions John expressed about surrogate mothers. He was an anomaly among intended parents, nonetheless, his extreme views exemplified some of the anxieties many surrogacy agencies, infertility doctors, and some intended parents had about the surrogate mothers. John implied that surrogate mothers were wily businesswomen who cared only about money, and the babies they birthed and gave up were insignificant in comparison. These manipulative women and their colluding husbands were not browbeaten and exploited; instead, they were scheming, calculating operators who misled and cheated intended parents who were erroneously characterized by the public at large as privileged individuals. According to John the real victims in this market exchange were the intended parents.

Though the surrogate mothers were disempowered by the way the market was organized, they were also the most feared agents. They were seen as exceedingly powerful individuals who could browbeat others, especially intended parents, involved in transnational surrogacy. They were projected as having so much power and potency because the entire labor process of making babies resided in their bodies and was in their control. Regardless of how skilled embryologists or infertility specialists were, without that mother's body and resolve to nurture that embryo into a fetus and then a baby, surrogacy would not be possible. Their consent had to be initiated, and their compliance to medical procedures and the entire labor process had to be enforced. The surrogate mothers were the most crucial element, the linchpin in India's reproduction assembly lines. It was because of their indispensability that they were so feared, and subsequently so heavily controlled by infertility doctors, surrogacy agencies, and recruiting agents. It was precisely this need for control that led infertility specialists to deliver many of the babies through caesarian sections. The surrogate mother was wrested of decision-making power in even the way she birthed the baby, or for that matter, what she did with her body afterward.

It was routine practice for some clinics to have the surrogate mothers produce pumped breast milk for the babies. One American client mother is an example; this woman had twins through surrogate mother Kailash in Gujarat. I have not interviewed this person and only have access to her self-representation on her blog:

> Everyone knows . . . Breast is better. Well, my breasts don't have any milk in them. . . . Kailash does have milk in her breasts and *I want it* . . . . Part of the surrogacy contract requires Kailash to provide breast milk for 15 days. After that, we can have more, but we need to negotiate the details. The first days in NICU [Neonatal Infant Care Unit], before we got here, I'm not sure what was happening on the breast milk front. I think nothing. Then I asked for it and Kailash started pumping. She was transferred 2 blocks to the hospital where the NICU was located for ease. I asked her to come down to NICU to pump every 2 hours, but somehow something was lost in the Gujarati-English translation. She did come, but only when my bossy nurse Sandiya called her down for feeding time. Love Sandiya! This was the easiest time for milk collection, yet somehow we were still just hitting maybe 4–5 pumping sessions per day . . . when the babies are

> eating 12 times. I realized *I needed to be managing Kailash and telling her what I wanted.* I erroneously assumed someone else directed her to pump every 2 hours and to deliver that milk to the babies. When we brought the babies back to the Rama [hotel] things got even worse. Now the milk needed to be delivered down the street. And the pump needed to be sterilized. Kailash is back at the Dr. Patel hospital where she gave birth. Every 2 hours, we need to fetch milk from Kailash and bring the pump back to the Rama for sterilization. Then the process begins again. Back and forth and forth and back. . . . I feel like a drug runner, or a gerbil on a treadmill. I'm almost ready to quit, but working on finding a runner to pay to do the back and forth. *Everything can be outsourced in India.* (Emphasis added)

While the client says she feels like a gerbil on a treadmill because she has to run back and forth to pick up breast milk, one can't help but wonder what Kailash must have gone through, to be summoned every so often to be milked on a machine to feed the American babies she had birthed, but were now too sacred to be held to her profane breasts.

In my three years of meeting with client parents, surrogacy agency owners, surrogate mothers, and infertility doctors, I had never grasped how a living person could be converted into a piece of property. It was this story that best illuminated for me how women were converted into machines, explicitly describing the complete takeover of a surrogate mother's body, converting her into rental property to manage her fecundity, control her birthing processes through caesarian surgeries, and finally, regulate her body's ability to sustain life through lactation, harvesting her milk in order to bottle feed the very babies she had just birthed. Markets in life operated by negating the life of some persons, specifically the women who signed up as surrogate mothers.

If it was important for some parents to have their babies nourished with breast milk, then why did they not just let the surrogate mothers breast-feed the babies? Why did they insist on breast pumps, continuing the process of extraction well past birth? It seemed that there was fear that the surrogate mother might feel tremendous love for the baby she had birthed and might have a possessive investment in that child. What if she wanted to keep the baby, or if she wanted to continue to be a part of the baby's life? It is precisely this love that a mother might feel for the child that caused revulsion for her.

Clients such as John and surrogacy agencies wondered what kind of woman she could be, to carry, labor, and birth a baby only to give it away for the sake of money? In John's words, these women "are in this for the money and could care less about anything else." What kind of unfeeling beast would not grow attached to the life she had nurtured within her? Or worse, what kind of monster mother was she to develop love for the life within her, yet give away something so sacred for profane money? Thus, the surrogate mother was implicitly and explicitly understood to be someone who was capable of anything. She has proven her depravity by engaging in contractual pregnancies and giving away a baby she has nurtured in her body for a trivial sum of money. Because of the labor she engaged in and the discounted wages she received, *she* became a dreaded social figure who had no morals. As a result, she could wreak havoc in intended parents' and the children's lives. John said he could "relay horror stories about how IPs [intended parents] have been burned" by such degenerate women and their conspiring husbands. According to some clients, surrogate mothers were the sorts of people who would continue to make financial and emotional demands, using the children they had birthed as tools to garner greater and greater economic and social benefits for themselves. They could potentially engage in "post-contractual opportunistic behavior" and emotionally blackmail clients into meeting their demands.[13]

Thus, as a preemptive move, infertility specialists and surrogacy agencies insisted that clients maintain strict standards of business transactions with surrogate mothers because if surrogacy became a form of gift exchange, there would be no protective barrier for clients. Sticking to the language of contract and operating as if the entire exchange was modulated only by the medium of money formed a barrier between the producer and the consumer. Clients protected themselves, their children, and their nuclear families from the *potential* social and financial demands they thought surrogate mothers would make on them if they maintained the ongoing social relationships characteristic of gift exchanges.

The surrogate mothers, however, had different ideas about the whole market exchange. From their perspective, they were morally superior gift givers of life; on the other hand, the intended parents were materialistic, immoral individuals who simply took life as if it was their birthright.

The Moral Value of Pregnancy and Childbirth

I was with Sita and her husband in their small living room in our very last meeting. She had just delivered twin baby boys prematurely and returned home. Sita looked unwell. She cried as she told me that one of the babies had died two days before. She was worried for the other baby who was fighting for his life in the Neonatal Intensive Care Unit (NICU). She felt that all the work that she had put in birthing the twin boys amounted to nothing. In the last days of her pregnancy Sita told the doctors that she could not feel one of the babies move but they did not take her seriously. They believed that she was making up stories because she wanted to birth the twins early in order to return home. The doctors eventually conducted her caesarian surgery three days later but it was too late. Sita was furious that they had ignored her.

Sita and her husband wanted to be with the surviving baby at the NICU but were not allowed there. She had never met her recipients. Two white men came to see the dying baby right at the very end, and she believed these were the intended parents. She and her husband sat together in their living room, far away from the NICU and devastated that *two* of their babies had died; a daughter at six months of age in the car accident almost two years earlier, and this little boy two days after birth. They did not know what awaited the surviving surrogated baby and prayed for a positive outcome for his life.

Sita's abandonment after delivery was the norm for surrogate mothers in Bangalore. Prabha never met her recipients even when they came to pick up the baby. Roopa longed to hold, or even receive pictures and news of, the baby she had birthed and given away three years earlier. She cooked elaborate meals to commemorate the surrogated baby's birthday, and hoped that wherever she was and whoever she was with, "her" little girl was happy and loved.

Twenty-seven-year-old Chandra, an *agarbathi* worker, mother of three daughters and prospective surrogate mother, was incensed. I was sitting with her and four other surrogate mothers on Kavita's floor and discussing how to deal with being separated from the surrogated baby when their time came. Kavita reiterated what she had said just days earlier, "The recipients pray to god that they may have a child. We surrogate mothers too pray, but to give us strength to give up that baby." She then continued that it was common practice in one of the infertility clinics in Bangalore to take away the baby the minute s/he was born. As the surrogate mother lay there, immobile and recovering from surgery, nurses and doctors whisked the baby out without telling her where the baby was going or who the prospective parents were. The women were not given the opportunity to hold the baby, and some mothers did not even know the sex of the baby they had birthed. At this point Chandra, who was receiving injections to become a surrogate mother, angrily interjected that she recognized why the intended parents might hesitate to bring the surrogate mother into their lives; she said that their love and appreciation could quickly turn sour if surrogate mothers called them too often after relinquishing the baby. They would wonder why the surrogate mother persisted in maintaining the relationship and would suspect that she wanted gifts or money from them. The relationship, then, would become a burden. Because Chandra did not want to bring such disgrace upon herself she would let the surrogated baby go. She continued:

> I have satisfaction (*atma trupti*)[14] in my own actions. I know that through my suffering I will have filled another home with a child. But what kind of

> people are these recipients? Can they ever have *atma trupti*? How do they face themselves and look that baby in the eye, knowing that they never allowed it to be even held in the arms of the mother (*hettha thai*)[15] who gave birth to him?

Chandra maintained that she would conduct herself honorably by giving up the baby. Her supreme sacrifice would help them fulfill their desire for a home filled with children. Though the loss of the baby would be hard on her, the knowledge that the intended parents' needs had been met would be a source of deep satisfaction for Chandra. She would have facilitated the perpetuity of their lineage (*vamsha*), which was extremely important for Hindu families. But she wondered how these people could live with themselves, what was their source of inner contentment, if they did not let the mother hold the surrogated baby? What did they gain by not sitting next to the surrogate mother, holding her hands, thanking her for all that she had done, and recognizing her and her family's efforts in fulfilling their desire for a baby? How could they embrace the surrogated baby and what did their love for the baby mean if they misrecognized and denigrated the efforts of the woman who had given birth to their baby? Through spectacular language, Chandra pointed to the sacrifices the surrogate mothers made, their matchless ability to create life value and give renewed hope to individuals who had once seemed so defeated. She castigated the various agents involved, though her ire here was reserved for those intended parents who failed to acknowledge the mother's power and sacrifice through oversight, or worse, through intention. Chandra did not want an alienated surrogacy experience. Instead, she wished for an engaged one. Such an experience did not necessarily entail maintaining lifelong bonds between her and the client parents, but rather, it was a process that was respectful of her efforts. Rather than be treated as a discardable woman, she wanted to be honored for her supreme sacrifice.

Like Chandra, many surrogate mothers recognized that their actions far superseded market exchanges. Even as they pointed to all the labor involved for which they had not been compensated, they also insisted that surrogacy was a gift. By moving this market exchange into the realm of the gift they reinserted their contributions to making the baby. No amount of money, many mothers claimed, came close to acknowledging the enormity of their maternal sacrifice and their supreme gift of life. Even as all the agents involved attempted to cast the mothers as atomized market agents and therefore fungible, the mothers reinserted themselves as moral actors who sacrificed so much to add so much to the world.

Conclusion

Discounted Life

At present India is the largest provider of surrogacy services in the world, surpassing even the United States, which held that esteemed ranking for much of our short history in transnational surrogacy. A large part of India's success has had to do with the sheer number of women who have signed on as surrogate mothers. They have been depicted as oppressed women who are easily exploitable. Yet upon meeting with seventy surrogate mothers in Bangalore, I realized that the overarching popular narrative of surrogate mothers as browbeaten, uninformed, easily duped villagers helplessly caught up in the web of global intimate industries was simply not true. Instead, they were wheelers and dealers, hustlers in a neoliberal global economy, attempting to get a secure foothold even as Bangalore's economy became increasingly fragile and unpredictable for urban working-class communities. They were out on the streets chatting with others during garment factory lunch breaks, in an attempt to locate the next big economic opportunity. They were ambitious; they wanted a better life for themselves and their families. Knowing that there was no cushion to break their economic fall, they built networks, sought information, and made clear-headed decisions about their finances even as they gambled with their bodies and health. Given their shrinking opportunities for economic mobility, they attempted to wring value from their bodies before their reproductive capacities faded as they entered their forties.

Each woman I spoke with felt her journey to surrogacy was unique, and it doubtless was. Yet standing back and listening to their stories, I discerned that their decisions did not come out of thin air. Their choices were made within a larger sociohistorical context , and this context was their own bodily entanglements with reproductive technologies, namely, sterilization, their personal histories as wage workers, mainly in Bangalore's garment sweatshops, and finally, Bangalore's underground market in babies.

It was not in their power to alter the endemic socioeconomic conditions that led to their precarity. Instead, what they saw around them were emergent markets in life. These new markets facilitated new ways to earn wages; they could receive money for something they had always done for free. That is, they could vend their reproductive capacities for wages. Yet they also recognized that Bangalore's reproductive assembly lines did not provide them with substantial and life-changing earnings. Nor were their labor experiences as surrogate mothers very empowering. They came to recognize that over the course of their stay at the dormitory, through their heavily medically mediated pregnancies and their caesarian deliveries, their labor, their bodies, and their lives were discounted. Some mothers attempted to change that by having greater control over marketing their reproductive abilities than was afforded to them in the current setup. They did not want to be discounted workers.

Surrogacy Cooperatives

On my last visit to Bangalore in the winter of 2011–12 Indirani invited me over to lunch at her home. Her sisters Kavita and Prabha, and Suma would be there too, she said. As we sat down cross-legged on the floor to eat platefuls of rice and lentils with mango pickle, the women launched into explaining why they wanted to meet with me. They wanted to start a surrogacy cooperative. They would recruit mothers who would not stay in a dormitory, but would reside in their own homes. The sisters and Suma would help the women attend their doctors' appointments, regulate diets as needed, and take all the precautions needed to sustain a high-risk pregnancy. After all, they said, they had been through the process themselves and knew what needed to be done. Once the mothers had delivered their babies they would be invited to be a part of the cooperative. On top

of paying women fair wages they would share the profits a
members, all of whom would be surrogate mothers.

Then they popped their question—given that I liv
States, could I find clients for them? I balked, because I ..
to become more entangled in these markets in life than I already was. .
promised the four women I would ask my contacts. Upon returning to Austin, Texas, I asked some of the intended parents I was in touch with if they would ever pursue surrogacy with a cooperative organized by current and former Indian surrogate mothers. While they agreed it was an interesting notion, they all balked at the idea of mothers with no "expert" supervision. No, they said. They would not work with a surrogate mothers' cooperative. To whom would they be held accountable? Could they trust these women with their tissue bits and cells meant to eventually become babies?

The surrogate mothers were complicit in converting their pregnancies into wage labor, but at the very least they wanted some control over the labor process. Though willing to sell their pregnancies they wanted to do so on their own terms. The intended parents too were similarly complicit in converting pregnancy into a form of wage labor and by extension the baby into a commodity, but they wanted restraints imposed on the surrogate mothers and wanted them to fulfill the terms of their labor contracts under conditions they, the clients, felt were acceptable to them. Their reason for doing so was not a simple distrust of the mothers. More important, they felt an immense, yet wobbly love for their forthcoming children, a possessive investment in these yet-to-emerge persons. If anything, an excess of love led to perversions in trust. And the actors to be mistrusted the most in the entire reproductive assembly line were the workers, the surrogate mothers.

Given the fraught nature of the transactions and the fact that these were dealings in human life, I could understand their fears. My understanding grew from one story that I kept hearing from Roopa almost each time we met; this was a story in which a surrogate mother had absconded during her pregnancy and kept the baby as her own.

Reclaiming Reproductive Labor

Roopa was excited. This was a meeting she had been longing to arrange for me. I got my chance when I returned to Bangalore in the winter of 2011–12 and I found myself on familiar ground: on Roopa's living room floor, but this time I was with twenty-five-year-old Shylaja who held her five-month-old baby daughter on her lap. Shylaja had had a very sheltered upbringing; she had never worked outside the home and her parents had arranged her marriage when she turned eighteen. But in all her years of marriage she was not able to get pregnant. She did not know whether she or her husband suffered from infertility because they were too poor for diagnoses or treatment. Instead they tried a variety of diets, undertook religious vows of fasting, went to temples to pray for a child, and performed Hindu rituals in order to successfully conceive. Nothing worked. Eventually, in desperation she took a vow (*harake*) to a deity in a small temple near her home. She would make the supreme sacrifice of giving away her firstborn child to a childless couple if only she and her husband were blessed with children in their lives. Yet even this did not have the desired effect, and the couple lived in the quiet, isolating despair of their childless marriage, all the while being secretly and openly disparaged by extended family members. She was not invited to marriages and other auspicious events because her very presence was a bad omen and she would bring the curse of infertility on newly married couples. Life was miserable, said Shylaja.

That was when she first heard of Mr. Shetty's COTW and surrogacy. She and her husband approached him. She was legally ineligible for surrogacy because by Indian law, surrogacy contracts are viable only with women who had previously birthed their own children. But as a surrogate mother Shylaja felt she could fulfill her religious vow that she would give away her firstborn child; this, she hoped, would remove the curse of infertility that plagued her marriage. Mr. Shetty was moved by the couple's plight and as was his common practice, he overlooked the legal requirements for recruiting surrogate mothers. He matched recipient clients for Shylaja. Embryos were prepared using sex cells that legally belonged to the clients; the embryo transfer went smoothly without a hitch, and soon Shylaja was pregnant. She loved being pregnant.

Midway through her pregnancy and her dormitory stay, however, trouble erupted. In May 2011 COTW came under investigation for alleged fraud, and the neighborhood council chairman took Mr. Shetty to court. Mr. Shetty asserted the accusations against him were politically and economically motivated because he had not paid the council chairman a bribe. No outsiders—researchers like me, journalists, or others—were allowed access, because the dormitory was in lockdown. The men who hung around COTW and were on Mr. Shetty's payroll, were now deployed as guards because they did not want the council chairman's henchmen to disrupt the dormitory. Shylaja said she felt that her life was in danger. She managed to escape to a Ganesha temple nearby one Tuesday evening, because Tuesdays were auspicious for temple goers and the temple tended to be crowded on that particular day of the week, especially in the evenings when devotees flooded in after work hours. She hid amongst the crowds and called her husband on her cell phone to pick her up. She was scared; the dormitory felt unsafe and she wanted to go home. Though she had never meant to do so, Shylaja did not return to COTW's premises.

Shylaja said she had no intention of breaking her surrogacy contract *or* her religious vow, but the longer she stayed away from the dormitory, the more she wanted to keep what she had begun considering as her firstborn child. She ended up giving birth to a baby girl vaginally, and together with her husband, was raising their baby girl. As she lovingly gathered the five-month-old baby in her arms, Shylaja declared she had gone through considerable hardship for seven years in order to have *her* child. It was her and her husband's right to nurture that baby in their loving home.

When I recounted this story to my friends and family in the United States, they were horrified. "But what about the client couple? They lost their baby," they exclaimed. I may have expressed similar concerns earlier, but after having met the surrogate mothers in Bangalore, I was unsure about who held parental rights over the baby. The persons who owned the sperm and eggs (both of which may well have been purchased in sperm and egg banks), or the woman who labored to make that baby? Could the moral right to raise the baby be decided solely on the basis of who had more money? Were women not allowed to change their minds? Whose suffering, and whose efforts mattered more? I have never met these client parents but could only imagine their longing for a child. But should Shylaja's and her husband's equally painful experiences with childlessness be discounted, and matter any less? To speak of reproductive rights, I realized, was leading to an impasse. Rights talk simply juxtaposed one person's rights over another person's rights. If there were winners, then there had to be losers.

Surrogacy and Reproductive Rights

Commenting on pregnancy and abortion in the United States, feminist philosopher Susan Bordo argues that women's, fetal, and fathers' rights jostle against each other. If a woman opts to terminate her pregnancy, fetal rights to life or her male partner's right to fatherhood are invoked. Whose rights, then, are to take precedence? Rights rhetoric in reproduction is posited as a zero sum game; a woman's choice to abort her pregnancy is potentially cast as a loss in fetal life or a denial of men's rights to father children.[1]

Very similar sorts of criticisms were made about clients who utilized transnational surrogacy services. Much like those "innocent and hapless" fetuses that are aborted by conniving women who want to control their reproductive destiny, surrogate mothers and clients were juxtaposed in a dialectic relation. Clients were accused of being rich individuals from the global north who oppressed impoverished, almost subjectless Third World women. Surrogate mothers, already destitute, desperate and without any kind of subjectivity, could only lose; and intended parents, already privileged and self-absorbed, could only gain through these global markets in life.

Interrogating the practices of transnational surrogacy through the lens of reproductive rights set intended parents against surrogate mothers. Such a perspective did not bring into consideration the challenges individuals in the global north and working-class Indian women faced in achieving their sexual, reproductive, and parental desires. Gay men, for example, faced insurmountable legal and social barriers to becoming fathers. Similarly, working-class Indian women who are surrogate mothers confronted overwhelming challenges in being affirmed as women, workers, wives, and mothers.

In direct contrast to those who castigate clients as self-indulgent, privileged individuals who oppress mothers, proponents of transnational surrogacy utilize the *very* same reproductive rights talk to posit that everyone's rights have been met, be they gay men, childless straight couples, or surrogate mothers who vend their reproductive abilities. The former get their desired children and the latter receive a life-altering sum of money. Surrogacy, they maintain, is a "win-win" situation. However, various critics point out that such an argument that everyone wins falsely sets up a field of universal, abstract individuals who are divorced from their specific social realities. Philosopher Alison Bailey says that to speak of rights meaningfully requires scrupulous attention to social milieu; that is, surrogate mothers' decisions must be firmly tethered to larger political, economic, and social processes.[2]

Indeed, in my research I do *just* that. Rather than falsely universalizing, my conversations with surrogate mothers in Bangalore revealed the different ways by which, because of their life circumstances, they chose to receive wages for pregnancy. And many women asserted that their transactions in markets in life were affirming in a way none of their labor experiences had been before.

In spite of all its nuances, the argument I have made so far is not so different from the "win-win" scenario proponents of transnational surrogacy posit. After all, no one coerced the intended parents and surrogate mothers to engage in transnational surrogacy. They opted to transact in markets in life of their own volition. They were independent, rational agents. And surrogate mothers were free to do what they wanted with their bodies. The bodies were theirs, and it was their choice to expend their reproductive capacities as they saw fit. My work shows that the rubric of reproductive rights is deeply entangled in choice talk, and because of that it loses its value for understanding the benefits or harms (*himse*, as some mothers called it) entailed in surrogacy. Instead, I suggest that reproductive justice is a far more effective framework to think through what transnational surrogacy means.

Surrogacy and Reproductive Justice

My research revealed that surrogacy *could* be a highly risky job. Almost none of the women I met in Bangalore visited gynecologists regularly, other than for their pregnancies, abortions, and tubal ligations. Upon becoming surrogate mothers, however, they were at the receiving end of the latest technologies the market had to offer. They received hormonal shots, their wombs were subjected to ultrasound scans, they were fed well-balanced, protein-rich diets, and their weight gain was carefully charted. They had the best prenatal care available, if one accepts these technological interventions as top-notch care. But such medical intervention was available to them only for the duration of their market pregnancies.

Toward the terminal end of their pregnancies, between weeks thirty-six and thirty-eight, many of the surrogate mothers I met were scheduled for caesarian deliveries, which allowed the doctors to plan the exact time and date of delivery in order to better organize their workdays. Because of the scheduled caesarians the surrogacy agency could calculate how many beds it had available in its dormitory, how many more new clients it could take on, and how many new mothers could be housed for new babies to be borne all over again. Moreover, by scheduling the births, the doctors and surrogacy agencies did not have to house the babies in neonatal units, coordinate care, and make crucial life or death decisions, if it came to that, for intended parents who had not yet arrived. The

babies were almost always delivered on sched
tions, giving new and ironic meaning to the te
tion. The intended parents too saw advantages
schedule. They could coordinate work and fa
nannies to care for the babies when they retu
plan their lives around the scheduled caesaria
rogate mothers. Biological time embodied in
growth of prenatal life, the preparedness of th
cervical softening, uterine contractions, and labor pain was converted into technological time. Clocks. Calendars. Work schedules.

But what of the surrogate mothers who were cut open? There is no published research on the long-term effects of caesarian sections that are routinely performed in the surrogacy industry in India, and many people believe these procedures are foolproof. The question arises, Are medical personnel so skilled at cutting open humans that there are no errors, and somehow each and every body miraculously heals itself by magically closing up the lacerations and wounds? Are bodily scars solely the surface marks of past histories? Are there no hypertrophic scarring, no painful keloids where gashes, slashes, and tears inflicted on the female body persist and painfully haunt the woman in the present? Nothing is known about these matters. And we know almost nothing about the long-term effects of repeatedly pumping synthetic sex hormones into women's bodies. Nor do we have definitive knowledge about the long-term health outcomes of babies born through IVF who are often preterm when delivered through caesarian sections.

It should come as no surprise to readers to learn that surrogate mothers did not perceive themselves as victims or as people brutalized in their employment in markets in life. It is almost an inherent human condition to make do with what one has, to perceive positive or negative developments as emerging from one's *own choice*, and to make meaning and see joy in everyday endeavors. To give in to the horrors of the precarity we face on a daily basis is to give up on life. Thus, so many of us, including Bangalore's surrogate mothers, operate in "states of denial."[3] Violence zed, atrocities accumulating so rapidly upon each other that ecome routine. The everyday degradation on the garment shop r, sterilization camps, the indignities of surveillance on sweatshops, mothers selling their babies so that they may feed older children dependent on them. All this is mundane. It is within these everyday depravities that women sold their ova and engaged in surrogacy. They believed that such economic engagements would pull them out of precariousness into a life of stability where they and their children would never have to make the choices they had made in their lives.

Women's choices to birth or not birth babies, to sell their reproductive services or not, to keep the children they birth or give them away—these decisions must be located in the economic and social realities that shape their lives. More than reproductive rights, reproductive justice provides a conceptual framework to pay attention not just to choice, but to the endemic social, political, and economic inequalities among different communities which shape individuals' abilities to access a good life. It is in this context that we can begin to appreciate Shylaja's prerogative in exercising her maternal rights to keep her baby. And it is only within this context that surrogacy cooperatives as envisioned by Indirani and her sisters make sense.

To fully grasp the concept of reproductive justice I turn to legal scholar Dorothy Roberts, who makes a crucial distinction between anti-discrimination and anti-subordination. She observes that anti-discrimination laws in the United States require intentional acts of discrimination by individual actors that result in real harm toward specific individuals. These laws tend to individualize both acts of prejudice and the inequalities that result because of deliberate acts. Instead of individual acts of overt discrimination by racist individuals, Roberts notes that racial habitus, social patterns, and social institutions perpetuate systemic discrimination against persons of color, which in turn compromises equality.

Roberts explains her case by focusing on black drug addicts who are pregnant and who are persecuted in far greater numbers than are white women in similar situations. In the first instance, there are few or no services that assist them in getting off drugs. And health services report them for having transferred illegal substances to their fetuses through their umbilical cords. Thus, the safest route for these women is to opt for abortions because carrying their pregnancies to term will, more often than not, result in their legal prosecution. Roberts notes that their access to reproductive choice—in this case, having babies—is severely compromised. By ignoring the women's right to birth children and by solely focusing on the harm individual mothers do to their babies (because there *are* negative effects on fetuses when mothers use restricted substances during their pregnancies), Roberts says the state actively propagates black women's subordination. She explains that by

> legitimizing fetal rights enforcement, the prosecution of crack-addicted mothers diverts public attention from social ills such as poverty, racism, and a misguided national health policy—implying instead that shamefully high black infant mortality rates are caused by the bad acts of individual mothers. Poor black mothers thus become the scapegoats for the black community's ill health. Punishing them assuages any guilt the nation might feel at the sight of an underclass with infant mortality at rates higher than those in some less developed countries.[4]

She proposes that laws should attend to anti-subordination; the equal protection clause must function to "dismantle racial hierarchy by eliminating state action or inaction that effectively preserves black subordination."[5]

Extending Roberts's argument to surrogate mothers in India, I maintain that like anti-discrimination laws, the legal, political, and medical processes involved in surrogacy are not meant to harm individual women. On the contrary, markets in life are believed to further everyone's, including working-class women's, rights. These markets are perceived to be open and fair, with full respect for women's autonomy. Thus, no one compels women to enter into surrogacy, and it is their choice to use their bodies as they wish. The political and economic capacity of the neoliberal Indian state to address inequalities and redistributive justice has been steadily decreasing. Under these circumstances, individual well-being can only be advanced in the market. The role of the state is limited to providing the institutional framework by furthering property rights and developing legal structures, to facilitate market practices. The state enables the market, and the market empowers women.

Yet an examination of social beliefs regarding women's worth, their labor options, and the increasingly untenable economic situations working-class women and their families face leads to a very different conclusion regarding transnational surrogacy. The Indian state cannot stand mute on the question of structured class and gendered inequalities, and innocently believe that establishing stringent market conditions in commercial surrogacy will somehow meet the needs of the working-class women who serve as surrogate mothers. Instead, it must consider social patterns and institutions that perpetuate women's subordinate status in society. These sorts of considerations might remain incomprehensible to state actors, given the long histories of reproductive interventions on women's bodies as evinced by the continued, indiscriminate sterilization of working-class women that continues to the present day, where women still die in mass sterilization camps. Government reports show that between 2003 and 2012, 1,434 women died through botched sterilization procedures, which averages to 12 deaths every month in that decade.[6]

Within this context of sterilization abuse, shrinking access to health care because of neoliberal privatization as I discuss in chapter 1, and the complete absence of affordable infertility services for the indigent in India, it is a travesty to posit that transnational surrogacy furthers reproductive justice. Transnational surrogacy may afford working-class women the ability to earn some money, but how do these markets in life facilitate their attempts to build long-lasting social and political capital, and lead dignified lives? If these are life-affirming developments, as the mothers *themselves* maintain, then why do they not wish similar "career"

choices for their daughters? It may just be that t
like the client parents, desire that their children l
tact sense of dignity and physical integrity, whicl
been unable to achieve in their lifetime.

Reproductive justice pushes us to consider "tl
lived experiences at home, at work, in school, in be
or any other place where they expend their creative
alter power relations in their favor."[7] If reproductive justice is to prevail, women must have access to comprehensive health care, where their nuclear and extended family members' health and medical needs are met, in order for them to live full and satisfying lives. And crucially, reproductive justice cannot prevail without an acute consciousness of social hierarchies that can only be confronted with the force of a critical mass of actors working in tandem with each other, across various social strata. If and when these conditions are met, then transnational surrogacy has the *potential* to be a part of reproductive justice.

In conclusion, I want to answer a question Roopa asked me when we first met. She had eyed me suspiciously and inquired who I was and why I wanted to study surrogacy. Was I a journalist? Would I take their photographs, and why did I want to record everything on a digital recorder? Very intimidated, in my stuttering Kannada I explained to Roopa that I was a sociologist and I wanted to write a book. I did not think surrogacy was good or bad, but I believed the industry was exploitative because middlemen made a killing. And no, I did not think surrogate mothers or commissioning parents were immoral. All I wanted was to learn why women became surrogate mothers. Roopa's face had lit up, "You mean you're writing a history book of these times. When my daughter grows up she can read your book and learn how hard I've worked to raise her. These past few years haven't been easy."

If Roopa were to ask me the same question now I would answer her differently. I would tell her that I am a proponent of surrogacy *if* working-class Indian women like her are treated with the dignity, respect, and honor they so desperately desire. I am a proponent too if sur-

[obscured]others have a choice in becoming pregnant in ways they choose, [obscured]ng to use their own eggs or clients' genetic materials. The mothers need to be able to opt out or into procedures such as transvaginal ultrasounds. They should have the choice to stay at home with their own families or live in dormitories. The mothers must be allowed to birth babies in ways they choose rather than being systematically cut open preterm. And if they desire to breast-feed the babies they birth, they must be allowed to do so. They need to receive wages or other forms of compensation that they find equitable and just. And if the mothers wish, the intended parents need to work at maintaining ongoing social relationships with them. If and when surrogate mothers are treated as full human beings, with respect for their emotional, physical, and intellectual well-being, their sense of self, dignity, and body intact, then I am an advocate of commercial transnational surrogacy.

NOTES

INTRODUCTION

1 David Jones, "The Designer Baby Factory: Eggs from Beautiful Eastern Europeans, Sperm from Wealthy Westerners and Embryos Implanted in Desperate Women," *Daily Mail*, May 4, 2012, accessed on November 18, 2013, http://www.dailymail.co.uk/news/article-2139708/The-designer-baby-factory-Eggs-beautiful-Eastern-Europeans-Sperm-wealthy-Westerners-And-embryos-implanted-desperate-women.html.

2 I use the terms *commissioning parents*, *intended parents*, *client parents*, and *recipients* to refer to those individuals who receive and raise the surrogated babies as their own. All these terms are fraught and none are appropriate. Does it make any sense to continue to call clients "intended" parents when their surrogated baby is a three-year-old toddler? Socially, emotionally, and intellectually they have moved far from simply expressing intent, and are deeply enmeshed in the tasks of parenting that include cleaning, holding, being annoyed, and laughing with the young ones in their lives. Yet given that we're talking about the exchange of money for pregnancy and newborn, often premature babies, I continue to use these terms while fully appreciating that the "intended" parents engage in full-on, day-in-day-out parenting once they take the surrogated babies home; their parenting has nothing to do with intent but with everyday, practical life.

3 Six of these interviews were conducted by Caitlyn Collins, Ph.D. candidate in Sociology at UT-Austin.

4 Infertility is defined as a reproductive age couple's inability to get pregnant in spite of regular intercourse over a year without contraception, and is seen to affect close to 15 percent of the world's population. See Effy Vayena, Patrick J. Rowe, and P. David Griffin, eds., *Current Practices and Controversies in Assisted Reproduction* (Geneva: WHO, 2002). Moreover, surrogacy in the United States has been an absolutely central way by which gay fathers too have been able to bring children into their lives and families. Most of the gay couples come from the West, rather than countries like South Korea, Japan, or India.

5 Susan Markens, *Surrogate Motherhood and the Politics of Reproduction* (Berkeley: University of California Press, 2007), 180–181.

6 Sharmila Rudrappa, "Outsourcing Labor: Transnational Surrogacy in India," in *Research in the Sociology of Work*, vol. 20 of *Gender and Sexuality in the*

Workplace, ed. Christine Williams and Kirsten Dellinger (Howard House, U.K.: Emerald Group Publishing Limited, 2010), 253–285.

7 Amrita Pande, "Transnational Commercial Surrogacy in India: Gifts for Global Sisters?" *Reproductive BioMedicine Online* 23 (2011): 618–625. There is no real data and different profit projections are made. One source notes that in 2006 an estimated 500,000 international travelers went to India specifically for its health care services, generating roughly $600 million in revenue, which is a fraction of the $150 billion worldwide market. Alan Naditz, "Healthcare Tourism: Opportunities for India," *Telemedicine and e-Health* 14, no. 3 (April 2008): 207. Regardless of what their estimates are, many commentators agree that India is the leading provider of surrogacy services to individuals around the world (Judy Norsigian, personal communication, October 2013).

8 http://icmr.nic.in/icmrnews/art/MHA_circular_July%209.pdf. Accessed on May 2, 2015.

9 Sharmila Rudrappa, "What to Expect When You're Expecting: Consuming Parenthood through Surrogacy in India," special issue titled "Intimate Industries: Restructuring (Im)Material Labor in Asia," ed. Rhacel Parreñas, Rachel Silvey, and Hung Cam Thai, *positions: asia critique* 24, no. 1 (2016). Also see Daisy Deomampo, "Gendered Geographies of Reproductive Tourism," *Gender & Society* 27, no. 4 (2013): 514–537; Daisy Deomampo, "Transnational Surrogacy in India: Interrogating Power and Women's Agency," *Frontiers: A Journal of Women Studies* 34, no. 3 (2013): 167–188.

10 Egg donors too are usually anonymous.

11 Marcia Inhorn, "Globalization and Gametes: Reproductive 'Tourism,' Islamic Bioethics, and Middle Eastern Modernity," *Anthropology and Medicine* 18, no. 1 (2011): 90.

12 See Shellee Colen, "Like a Mother to Them: Stratified Reproduction and West Indian Childcare Workers and Employers in New York," in *Conceiving the New World Order: The Global Politics of Reproduction*, ed. Faye D. Ginsburg and Rayna Rapp (Berkeley: University of California Press, 1995), 78; Eileen Boris and Rhacel Parreñas, eds., *Intimate Labors: Cultures, Technologies, and the Politics of Care* (Stanford: Stanford University Press, 2010); Sharmila Rudrappa, "Working India's Reproductive Assembly Line: Surrogacy and Reproductive Rights?" *Western Humanities Review* 66, no. 3 (2012): 77–101.

13 Michal Nahman, "Nodes of Desire: Romanian Egg Sellers, 'Dignity' and Feminist Alliances in Transnational Ova Exchanges," *European Journal of Women's Studies* 15, no. 2 (2008): 65–82; Elly Teman, *Birthing a Mother: The Surrogate Body and The Pregnant Self* (Berkeley: University of California Press, 2010); Sharmila Rudrappa, "5: Gay Fathers and Indian Surrogate Mothers," in *Globalized Fatherhood*, ed. Marcia Inhorn, Wendy Chavkin, and Jose-Alberto Navarro (Oxford: Berghahn Books, 2015).

14 Rayna Rapp, "Reproductive Entanglements: Body, State, and Culture in the Dys/regulation of Childbearing," *Social Research* 78, no. 3 (2009): 1–52.
15 Pande, 2011.
16 Ellen Lewin, *Gay Fatherhood: Narratives of Family and Citizenship in America* (Chicago: University of Chicago Press, 2009).
17 Rudrappa, 2014.
18 Amrita Pande, "Not an 'Angel,' Not a 'Whore': Surrogate as 'Dirty' Workers in India," *Indian Journal of Gender Studies* 16, no. 2 (2009): 141–173.
19 Melinda Cooper, *Life as Surplus* (Seattle: University of Washington Press, 2008).
20 Nikolas Rose, *The Politics of Life Itself: Biomedicine, Power, and Subjectivity in the Twenty-First Century* (Princeton: Princeton University Press, 2006); Kaushik Sunder Rajan, *Biocapital* (Durham: Duke University Press, 2006).
21 Catherine Waldby, *The Visible Human Project: Informatic Bodies and Posthuman Medicine* (London: Routledge, 2000), 19.
22 Barbara Katz Rothman first introduced the term "reproductive assembly line" in *Recreating Motherhood* (New Brunswick, NJ: Rutgers University Press, 2000). She writes that when we begin to perceive products of conception "as just that, as products, we begin to treat them as we do any other product, subject to similar scrutiny and standards. As babies and children become products, mothers become producers, pregnant women the unskilled workers on a reproductive assembly line" (2000: 6). Speaking presciently about the legal, medical, psychological, and political recreation of modern motherhood, she notes that, "Babies, at least healthy white babies, are very precious products these days. Mothers, rather like South African diamond miners, are cheap, expendable, not-too-trustworthy labor necessary to produce the precious product" (2000: 39).
23 Arlie Hochschild, *The Outsourced Self: Intimate Life in Market Times* (New York: Metropolitan Books, 2012).
24 Boris and Parreñas, 2010: 5.
25 Rhacel Parreñas, Hung Thai, and Rachel Silvey, "Introduction," special issue titled "Intimate Industries: Restructuring (Im)Material Labor in Asia," *positions: asia critique positions: asia critique* 24, no. 1 (2016).
26 In her work on transnational adoption, Laura Briggs (2012) shows that not just child care, but child bearing for others is also a form of globalized intimate labor. Transnational adoption, whereby families from the West seek babies from Guatemala, China, or Russia, for example, depends on the reproductive labor of mothers in these southern countries to fulfill their familial needs. *Laura Briggs, Somebody's Children: The Politics of Transracial and Transnational Adoption* (Durham: Duke University Press, 2012).
27 See Arjun Appadurai, ed., *The Social Life of Things: Commodities in Cultural Perspective* (Cambridge: Cambridge University Press, 1986); Pierre Bourdieu, *The Logic of Practice* (Stanford: Stanford University Press, 1990); Arlie Hochschild, *The Managed Heart: The Commercialization of Human Feeling* (Berkeley:

University of California Press, 1983); Marcel Mauss, *The Gift: The Form and Reason for Exchange in Archaic Societies* (London: Routledge, 1990); Karl Polanyi, *The Great Transformation: The Political and Economic Origins of Our Times* (Boston: Beacon Press, 1971); Gayle Rubin, "Traffic in Women: Notes on the 'Political Economy' of Sex," in *Deviations: A Gayle Rubin Reader* (Durham: Duke University Press, 2011); Marilyn Strathern, *The Gender of the Gift: Problems with Women and Problems with Society in Melanesia* (Berkeley: University of California Press, 1990).

28 Nancy Scheper-Hughes and Loic Wacquant, *Commodifying Bodies* (London: Sage, 2003); Catherine Waldby and Robert Mitchell, *Tissue Economies: Blood, Organs, and Cell Lines in Late Capitalism* (Durham: Duke University Press, 2006). More recently, sociologist Rene Almeling asks how and why human eggs come to be seen as gifts, whereas sperm are commodities. Rene Almeling, *Sex Cells: The Medical Market for Eggs and Sperm* (Berkeley: University of California Press, 2011).

29 Anthropologist Christopher Gregory explains that commodities that circulate in markets are characterized by exchanges "of alienable things between transactors who are in a state of reciprocal independence." Contrarily, gift exchange is marked by the exchange "of inalienable things between transactors who are in a state of reciprocal dependence." Christopher Gregory, *Gifts and Commodities* (London: Academic Press, 1982),12.

CHAPTER 1. REPRODUCTIVE INTERVENTIONS

1 I take the phrase "demographic deluge" from Sanjay Gandhi. Cited in Davidson R. Gwatkin, "Political Will and Family Planning: India's Emergency Experience," *Population and Development Review* 5, no. 1 (1979): 29–59. Sanjay Gandhi, second son of Indira Gandhi, was the force behind sterilization abuse in India between 1975 and 1977.

2 Lawrence Cohen's research on the market in kidneys in the southern Indian city of Chennai is especially instructive. Borrowing the term bioavailability from medicine to describe how foreign, transferred tissue materials become available to the host body, Cohen (2008) explains how entire populations are made bioavailable for the removal of kidneys to be implanted into others. That is, geographical zones appear, where bodies present themselves with harvestable kidneys ready to be transplanted into others' bodies. He shows that most of those who sell their kidneys are women, and most of these women have undergone sterilization. The prior operability of these individuals makes them open for future operations. Lawrence Cohen, "Operability, Bioavailability, and Exception," in *Global Assemblages: Technology, Politics, and Ethics and Anthropological Problems*, ed. Aihwa Ong and Stephen Collier (Oxford: Blackwell, 2008).

3 Abhishek Singh, Reuben Ogollah, Faujdar Ram, and Saseendran Pallikadavath, "Sterilization Regret among Married Women in India: Implications for the Indian

National Family Planning Program," *International Perspectives on Sexual and Reproductive Health* 38, no. 4 (2012): 187–195. Between 55 percent and 63 percent of married women opted for sterilization in 2005–06 in Andhra Pradesh, Karnataka, and Tamil Nadu, which have the lowest fertility rates in the country. The median age at sterilization was particularly low in Andhra Pradesh (23.3 years), Karnataka (23.9 years), and Tamil Nadu (24.9 years). See *National Family Health Survey (NFHS-3)*,1 (Mumbai: IIPS, 2005–06).

4 Almost two-thirds of the women on the pill received their most recent supply from the privatemedical sector, which is also the most common source for condoms. See International Institute for Population Sciences (IIPS) and Macro International, *National Family Health Survey (NFHS-3), India 2005–06: Karnataka* (Mumbai: IIPS, 2008).

5 Janaki Nair writes that Mysore boasted of an impressive list of firsts among all princely states. "Not only did it have the first Representative Assembly (1881) and the first Legislative Council (1907), it was the first to use electric power to illuminate cities (Bangalore in 1905), to establish a state bank (1913), to start a university (1916), to found a Chamber of Commerce, (1916), to initiate the first programme of reservation for Backward Classes (1918), to set up a Serum Institute (1929), to fund birth control clinics for the general public (1930), to send a trade commissioner to London (1930), and to run an Administrative Training Institute for Indian princes. Its policy of state aid to industries became the envy of South India, inasmuch as it paved the way for the location of major public sector industries in the immediate post-independence period. Above all it introduced many innovative administrative measures aimed at redressing caste and gender inequalities, which earned Mysore the praise of feminists and other activists in British ruled territories" (2008, 211). See Janaki Nair, "'Imperial Reason,' National Honour, and New Patriarchal Compacts in Early Twentieth-century India," *History Workshop Journal* 66, no. 1 (2008): 208–226.

6 Newspapers from 1930, though, claim there were four. For example, under the headline, "State Birth Control Clinics: Innovation in Mysore," on September 20, 1930 the *Glasgow Herald* notes: "Reuter's Agency learns that a step, which is probably without precedent in India, has been taken by the Government of the Indian State of Mysore, which has given official approval to the establishment at the four principal hospitals in the State of State birth control clinics. The innovation is the outcome of the conviction, as a result of his professional experience, of the senior surgeon in Mysore—himself an Indian—that facilities for instruction in birth control are called for in the interests of many women in the State." http://news.google.com/newspapers?nid=2507&dat=19300920&id=2XVDAAAAIBAJ&sjid=caUMAAAAIBAJ&pg=5383,2886703. Accessed on June 27, 2014. The effectiveness of these clinics is questionable; in a letter to Margaret Sanger dated February 23, 1935, Edith How-Martyn writes that these clinics were not working satisfactorily. *The Margaret Sanger Papers, Status of birth control in*

India, 1930s. http://editorsnotes.org/projects/sanger/notes/187/. Accessed on June 27, 2014.

7 For population control during colonialism, see Sarah Hodges, *Contraception, Colonialism and Commerce: Birth Control in South India, 1920–1940* (Burlington: Ashgate, 2008).

8 A good overview of postindependence developments is provided by Rosanna Ledbetter, "Thirty Years of Family Planning in India," *Asian Survey* 24, no. 7 (July 1984), 736–758. The nation's First Five Year Plan (1951–56) made interventions in population growth an explicit part of economic development strategies by allocating Rs. 6.5 million to the newly created Indian Family Planning Programme in 1952. However, only 152,677 sterilizations were achieved by 1961. Ledbetter notes that the Third Plan (1961–66) aimed for better results; in 1961 allocations to the Family Planning Programme increased to Rs.250 million and every kind of birth control, except for the pill, which had just been introduced in the United States, was implemented (1984: 740). Also see Mohan Rao's excellent book, *From Population Control to Reproductive Health: Malthusian Arithmetic* (New Delhi: Sage, 2005).

9 See Matthew Connelly, "Population Control in India: Prologue to the Emergency Period," *Population and Development Review* 32, no. 4 (2006): 639–667. Also his absolutely compelling *Fatal Misconception: The Struggle to Control World Population* (Cambridge: Harvard University Press, 2009). Connelly says that some of these population control "activists" were driven by racial concerns regarding the fertility of women of color across the world, including the United States.

10 Connelly, 2006: 630. Matthew Connelly writes that Lyndon B. Johnson "publicly declared that less than five dollars invested in population control was worth a hundred dollars directly invested in economic growth. Without necessarily understanding the basis for this claim, the president had signed off on the idea that children in poor countries could be a net liability. Even more important, he now insisted on personally approving every new food shipment to India, typically a month's supply in a policy that came to be known as the 'short leash'" (2006: 647).

11 IUDs were difficult to use because of the significant pain involved in insertion; women needed to receive local anesthesia in order to have a trained physician first dilate the cervix to insert the IUD. Moreover, these IUDs caused pelvic inflammatory disease (PID) in women because the tail of the device hung out of the cervix and wicked infection, causing bacteria to enter into the body. Removing IUDs was equally problematic because the uterine walls could get scratched or perforated.

12 Cited in Connelly, 2009: 202.

13 See Connelly, 2006: 657.

14 By the end of 1966, 810,000 women had IUDs (Ledbetter, 1984). In 1967 over 910,000 women were inserted with IUDs, but that number fell to 479,000

women by 1969. In spite of the disciplinary action against revenue officers for bringing in too few women and government physicians for "underperforming" because they did not meet targets, *and* the incentives offered to IUD "acceptors," women were unwilling to take on the risks that included painful prolonged pelvic infections, ectopic pregnancies, and eventually, infertility. See James G. Chadney, "Family Planning: India's Achilles' Heel?" *Journal of Asian and African Studies* 22 (July 1987): 217.

15 India's economic problems were seen as so severe beginning in 1965, that between 1966 and 1969 then Prime Minister Indira Gandhi suspended the five-year plans in favor of annual budgets (Ledbetter, 1984).

16 A state-owned factory, Hindustan Latex Ltd. was established in 1966 in Trivandrum, Kerala, to produce condoms. The United States provided 2 million condoms annually but by the early 1970s India was producing enough to meet internal demand (Ledbetter, 1984: 742–3). When IUD acceptance declined, the number of condom acceptors increased from 465,000 to 961,000 persons annually in the late 1960s (Chadney, 1987: 222).

17 Singh et al., 2012.

18 Government employees were given five days' leave from work for accepting sterilization, and businesses were encouraged to participate in the program. Private companies too jumped into the fray. For example, Tata Group, an Indian multinational conglomerate, incentivized male workers to undergo vasectomies after the birth of a third child by offering Rs.250 plus numerous days of leave (Ledbetter, 1984: 743).

19 State employees such as postmen and village schoolteachers were urged to sell condoms to the public at subsidized rates; in the 1960s three condoms cost less than a penny (Ledbetter, 1984: 743).

20 Alan Guttmacher, cited in Connelly, 2009: 201.

21 Connelly, 2006.

22 See Chadney, 1987: 223. Davidson Gwatkin (1979) says the Kerala experiment is noteworthy because close to U.S. $11 was provided to sterilization acceptors, which was more than a month's salary for an unskilled worker. Maudlin and Sinding (1993) write that the district revenue collector of the Ernakulum District in Kerala led the camp effort; appeals for assistance went to the private sector, NGOs, and local leaders. The entire government sector was notified and asked to participate fully. Responsibilities for various tasks such as motivating people, recruiting doctors, and setting up the camps were delegated to various committees. W. Parker Maudlin and Steven W. Sinding, *Review of Existing Family Planning Policies and Programs: Lessons Learned* no. 50 (Population Council Working Papers, 1993).

23 Maudlin and Sinding, 1993: 32–33.

24 Gwatkin, 1979: 33.

25 My source is an online publication put out by the National Population Stabilization Fund, which is registered as an autonomous society with the Indian Ministry of Health and Family Welfare. http://www.jsk.gov.in/faq.asp#b24. Accessed on June 24, 2014.

26 Singh et al., 2012.

27 Dr. Madusudan Das at the Vani Vilas government hospital in Bangalore said that more than 2,800 sterilizations had been performed on women between 2008 and 2011 at the hospital, but none on men. B. K. Krithika, "Indian Men Leave Sterilization to Women," *UPI Next*, December 14, 2011, accessed on June 24, 2014. http://next.upi.com/archive/2011/12/14/Indian-men-leave-sterilization-to-wives/8001323840752/.

28 Various states had toyed with the idea of compulsory sterilization in the early 1970s; for example, Uttar Pradesh wanted to deny education to children who came from large families, and the government of Maharashtra wanted to incentivize sterilization by not providing state-sponsored loans and subsidies to families with more than three children. The central government of India declared these legislative moves to be unconstitutional and disallowed them (Gwatkin, 1979). The Emergency, however, changed all that.

29 Cited in Gwatkin, 1979: 35.

30 Of the 1,800 deaths registered, 900 were investigated, and 700 of them resulted in compensation payment (Gwatkin, 1979: 47).

31 Gwatkin, 1979: 48.

32 Singh et al., 2012.

33 Alaka Basu, "Family Planning and the Emergency: An Unanticipated Consequence," *Economic and Political Weekly* 20, no. 10 (1985): 422–425. Singh et al. (2012), however, attribute the shift from male to female sterilization to a number of other factors, including the development of laparoscopic techniques for female sterilization, misconceptions about the side effects of vasectomies, including the loss of libido, the expansion of women-centered development programs such as the World Bank-funded Reproductive and Child Health program, and a central government scheme that compensated women more than men for accepting sterilization.

34 http://www.jsk.gov.in/faq.asp#b24. Accessed on June 24, 2014.

35 Of the sterilized women, 22 percent have a primary school education; and 70 percent have at least a secondary education. See Bornali Dutta, Chandrashekar, and Sayeed Unisa, "Female Sterilization in India: A comparison of static and mobile services delivery," n.d., accessed on June 28, 2014. http://www.iussp.org/sites/default/files/event_call_for_papers/Female%20Sterilization%20in%20India_1.pdf.

36 Cecilia van Hollen notes that in 1986–87 Tamil Nadu far exceeded its IUD acceptor target goals; in fact, almost double the targeted percentage of women were inserted with IUDs. The numbers for the following year were equally good, with Tamil Nadu reaching 171.4 percent of its target. A large part of this can

perhaps be explained by the routine insertion of IUDs into women when they went to hospitals to give birth to their babies. According to a demographer van Hollen interviewed, in 1995 the goal of family planning in the state was that 70 percent of all the women leaving the hospital after childbirth had to be covered with some sort of family planning method, namely, an IUD or sterilization. See Cecilia Van Hollen, *Birth on the Threshold: Childbirth and Modernity in South India* (Berkeley: University of California Press, 2003).

37 See Amarjeet Sinha, *Indian Democracy and Well-Being: An Inquiry into the Persistence of Poverty in a Dynamic Democracy* (New Delhi: Rupa, 2005). Conversations with various gynecologists who had participated in sterilization programs indicate that Tamil Nadu first innovated this practice, which proved to be highly successful in running effective and well-attended sterilization camps. Seeing this success Karnataka followed suit. However, Maudlin and Sinding (1993) record that the practice of pulling revenue officers into "family planning" efforts began in Kerala with vasectomy camps in 1970.

38 Barge and Ramchander (1999) confirm what I'd learnt from my informal conversations with gynecologists in Bangalore over the course of 2011. They conducted a study of five sterilization camps in the central Indian state of Madhya Pradesh in 1995, all of which were set up in school buildings at a distance of 15–50 kilometers from the closest primary health center (PHC) because most clients were unwilling to travel to the PHC; 82 women were sterilized in these three camps. The facilities in the camps varied greatly. Running water was not available in the classrooms converted into temporary operation rooms and had to be stored in plastic containers for use during and after surgeries. Though highly competent, the doctors did not have time to sterilize the equipment between the laparoscopic surgeries. There were no electrical facilities in the camps, and the lights had to be powered by jeep batteries; candles, torches, and kerosene lanterns were used for additional lighting. They note that postoperative care of patients was negligible in the outreach camps. Sandhya Barge and Laksmi Ramchander, "Provider and Clients Interactions in Primary Health Care: A Case Study from Madhya Pradesh," in *Improving Quality of Care in India's Family Welfare Programme: The Challenge Ahead*, ed. Michael A. Koening and M. E. Khan (New York: Population Council, 1999), 92–116.

39 For example, a March 2008 government manual gives detailed instructions on how to set up a camp, recruit service providers, recruit and bus in sterilization acceptors, and institute infection prevention methods. It also provides a list of pharmaceutical products needed along with their side effects, and lists of potential infections and the management of medical emergencies such as cardiac arrests should they occur. See Family Planning Division, Ministry of Health and Family Welfare, Government of India, *Standard Operating Procedures for Sterilization Services in Camps* (New Delhi: Government of India, March 2008).

40 Deaths in sterilization camps are routine news, as evinced by the latest disaster when 20 women died, and at least 30 others were in critical condition after being operated on in a free sterilization camp in central India. The surgeon had performed surgeries on 83 women in less than five hours, far more than the numbers recommended. All the women had received cash incentives of up to $22 for their compliance to the medical procedure. See Annie Gowen, "Deaths Shine Light on 'Horrible' Conditions in India's Mass Sterilization Camps," *Washington Post*, November 12, 2014, accessed on January 11, 2015. http://www.washington-post.com/world/asia_pacific/ deaths-shine-light-on-horrible-conditions-in-indias-mass-sterilization-camps/2014/11/12/8c409a9d-fc2b-49d2–842d-419de320236b_story.html.

41 This section is a shortened, revised version of my earlier article, Rudrappa, 2010.

42 In 1960 the birth control pill was approved for contraceptive use in the United States. In 1965 the Supreme Court in the United States awarded married women the right to use birth control as a constitutional right to privacy. Five years later President Nixon signed into law Title X of the Public Health Service Act, which made contraceptives available to all women regardless of marital status. On January 22, 1973, the U.S. Supreme Court handed down its landmark decision in *Roe v. Wade*, recognizing the constitutional right to privacy and women's right to choose abortion. Centering mostly on individual privacy rights, in the past fifty years American women's abilities to temporarily or permanently halt their fertility has expanded in fits and starts.

43 Susan Kahn, *Reproducing Jews: A Cultural Account of Assisted Conception in Israel* (Durham: Duke University Press, 2000); Marcia Inhorn and Frank van Balen, eds., *Infertility Around the Globe: New Thinking on Childlessness, Gender, and Reproductive Technologies* (Berkeley: University of California Press, 2002).

44 Groesbeck P. Parham and Michael L. Hicks, "Racial Disparities Affecting the Reproductive Health of African American Women," *Medical Clinics of North America* 89 (2005): 935–943.

45 Markens, 2007: 180–181.

46 Liza Mundy, *Everything Conceivable: How Assisted Reproduction Is Changing Men, Women, and the World* (New York: Anchor, 2007), 21.

47 From http://www.cdc.gov/art/. Accessed on March 24, 2014.

48 Since then the Bourn Hall Clinic has opened affiliated branches in Gurgaon, northern India, Kochi, southern India, and Dubai, UAE.

49 http://www.marketresearch.com/Marketdata-Enterprises-Inc-v416/Fertility-Clinics-Infertility-Services-2403343/. Accessed on March 24, 2014. Some commentators note that companies that make fertility drugs underwrite the market expansion of assisted reproductive technologies. For example, Ares Serono, a biotechnology company headquartered in Geneva, Switzerland, and lead supplier of fertility medication, notably Pergonal, funded the establishment of Drs. Edward's and Steptoe's Bourn Hall Clinic. Charis Thompson, *Making*

Parents: The Ontological Choreography of Reproductive Technologies (Cambridge: MIT Press, 2005), 233.

50 Reports on the number of infertility clinics in India vary from a low of 500 to the preposterous figure of 3,000 . See Rashmi K. Pratap, "IVF: Baby Boom," *Outlook Business*, October 15, 2011, accessed on March 24, 2014. http://business.outlookindia.com/printarticle.aspx?278530. The acronym NARI (National Association for Assisted Reproduction in India) ironically spells out the Hindi word for "woman." The U.K. based *Daily Mail* reports the exaggerated statistic. Nita Bhalla and Mansi Thapliyal, "Inside a 'Baby-Making Factory': How the Rent-a-Womb Industry Became India's Latest Booming Industry," *Daily Mail*, September 30, 2013, accessed on March 24, 2014. http://www.dailymail.co.uk/news/article-2439297/How-IVF-treatment-Indias-latest-booming-industry.html.

51 http://www.nobelprize.org/nobel_prizes/medicine/laureates/2010/press.html. Accessed on March 24, 2014.

52 Helena Ragone, *Surrogate Motherhood: Conception in the Heart* (Boulder: Westview Press, 1994); Lisa Ikemoto, "Eggs as Capital: Human Egg Procurement in the Fertility Industry and the Stem Cell Research Enterprise," *Signs* 34, no. 4 (2009): 763–781; Ruby Lee, "New Trends in Global Outsourcing of Commercial Surrogacy: A Call for Regulation," *Hastings Women's Law Journal* 20 (Summer 2009): 275–300.

53 Rapp, 2009.

54 Various newspaper accounts note that Dr. Mukhopadhyay published his research in Indian journals and was disciplined by the state government. He was prevented from presenting his work at scientific conferences and was eventually transferred in 1981 to the ophthalmology department, an area in which he had no expertise. He committed suicide later that year. See Aditya Bharadwaj, "Conception Politics: Medical Egos, Media Spotlights, and the Context of Test-Tube and Firsts in India," in *Infertility Around the Globe: New Thinking on Childlessness, Gender, and Reproductive Technologies*, ed. Marcia C. Inhorn and Frank van Balen (Berkeley: University of California Press, 2002), 319.

55 Ibid., 323

56 The most common practice in surrogacy is to use third-person donor eggs, instead of surrogate mothers' eggs. Part of the reasoning is that women who "donate" eggs are seen as different from are women who hire themselves out as surrogate mothers. That is, egg donors are from a more desirable gene pool; although surrogate mothers' genes do not matter, their compliance with medical intervention does (Rudrappa, 2010). But crucially, the surrogate mother has far fewer legal rights over the newborn if she has no genetic connection to the baby.

57 Thompson, 2005: 8.

58 This section is an updated version of an earlier publication, Rudrappa, 2012.

59 Sayeed Unisa, "Childlessness in Andhra Pradesh, India: Treatment-Seeking and Consequences," *Reproductive Health Matters* 7, no. 13 (1999): 54–64; Inhorn and

van Balen, 2002; Ruth Deech, "Reproductive Tourism in Europe," *Global Governance* 9 (2003): 425–432; Anjali Widge, "Seeking Conception in India: Experience of Urban Indian Women with In-Vitro Fertilisation," *Patient Education and Counseling* 59, no. 3 (2005): 226–233.

60 Colen, 1995: 84.

61 Susan Greenhalgh, ed., *Situating Fertility: Anthropology and Demographic Inquiry* (Cambridge: Cambridge University Press, 2005). Also see Unisa, 1999.

62 Marcia Inhorn and Daphna Birenbaum-Carmeli, "Assisted Reproductive Technologies and Culture Change," *Annual Review of Anthropology* 37 (October 2008): 177–196.

63 Marcia Inhorn and Daphna Birenbaum-Carmeli, "Assisted Reproductive Technologies and Culture Change," *Annual Review of Anthropology* 37 (October 2008): 177–196.

64 I use the phrase "cross-border reproductive care" (Inhorn and Gurtin, 2011; Inhorn and Patrizio, 2012) rather than the more commonly used "reproductive tourism" because, far from the relaxation and rejuvenation suggested by the term "tourism," those seeking reproductive attention are stressed about egg retrievals, sperm deposits, and making decisions about egg donors or surrogate mothers. They are dealing with unfamiliar legal regimes and cultures of medical practice that are deeply unsettling rather than relaxing. See Marcia C. Inhorn and Zeynep B. Gurtin, "Cross-Border Reproductive Care: A Future Research Agenda," *Reproductive BioMedicine Online* 23 (2011): 665–676. Also see Marcia C. Inhorn and Pasquale Patrizio, "The Global Landscape of Cross-Border Reproductive Care: Twenty Key Findings for the New Millennium," *Current Opinion in Obstetrics & Gynecology* 24, no. 4 (2012): 158–163.

65 Arthur L. Greil, Julia McQuillan, Michele Lowry, and Karina M. Schreffler, "Infertility Treatment and Fertility-Specific Distress: A Longitudinal Analysis of a Population-Based Sample of U.S. Women," *Social Science and Medicine* 73, no. 1 (July 2011): 87–94. Also see Gay Becker, Martha Castrillo, Rebecca Jackson, and Robert D. Nachtigall, "Infertility among Low-Income Latinos," *Fertility and Sterility* 85 (2005): 882–887.

66 Parham and Hicks, 2005.

67 Amelia Gentleman, "India Nurtures Business of Surrogate Motherhood," *New York Times*, March 10, 2008. http://www.nytimes.com/2008/03/10/world/asia/10surrogate.html. Accessed on July 2, 2009.

68 Roberto Matorras, "Reproductive Exile versus Reproductive Tourism," *Human Reproduction* 20, no. 12 (2005): 3571.

69 The WTO is an intergovernmental organization established in 1995 and based in Geneva to promote global free trade. Its membership consists of about 150 nation-states. It provides a forum for states to address issues relating to trade by bringing together state representatives once every two years and serves as a neutral third party to settle disputes between nation-states. Between 1980 and

2000 the total monetary value of exports in services increased by more than 400 percent, from $364 billion to $1.4 trillion, which brought trade in services to WTO's attention, leading to the General Agreement on Trade in Services, or GATS. See Ian S. Mutchnick, David T. Stern, and Cheryl A. Moyer, "Trading Health Services across Borders: GATS, Markets, and Caveats," *Health Affairs* (January 2005). Observers note that the 2000 GATS "imposes severe constraints on government's ability to protect environmental, health, consumer, and other public interest standards. It restricts government funding of public works, municipal services, and social programs. It guarantees access of private service corporations to domestic markets in all sectors. Every service imaginable is on the table." See Meneleo D. Litonjua, "International Free Trade, the WTO, and the Third World/Global South," *Journal of Third World Studies*, 27, no. 2 (2010): 60.

70 Andrea Wittaker, "Pleasure and Pain: Medical Travel in Asia," *Global Public Health* 3, no. 3 (2008): 271–290.

71 K. B. Saxena, "Trade in Health Services: Implications for People's Health," *Social Change* 41, no. 2 (2011): 183–213.

72 "India Slashes Health Budget, Already among World's Lowest: Report," December 23, 2014, accessed on December 25, 2014. http://www.ndtv.com/article/india/india-slashes-health-budget-already-among-world-s-lowest-report-638877?site=classic.

73 Annually, more than 100,000 mothers die in India during childbirth, which amounts to one maternal death every five minutes. Infant mortality rates are still very high, at 70 per live births. See Ramani RV and Mavalankar Dileep, "Health System in India: Opportunity and Challenges for Improvements," *Journal of Health Organization and Management* 20, no. 6 (2006): 560–572. These developments lead some scholars, notably Unger et al., to provocatively ask whether there is a causal link between current health policies and stagnating maternal and infant mortality. Unger et al. note that privatization of health care can be seen from 1985 onwards, when the United States withheld its contribution to the WHO on the basis of the argument that the provision of comprehensive health care in public services was abysmal. Unger et al. say that the academic community endorsed this new perspective, "which generated a wealth of publications depicting public health care provision as inefficient, bureaucratic and unresponsive. These publications actively promoted the privatisation of health care via the purchaser–provider split, autonomous management of public hospitals, contracting out of services, private financing initiatives and managed care, dressed as 'scientific guidance'" (2009: 92). See Jean-Piere Unger, Patrick Van Dessel, Kasturi Sen, and Pierre De Paepe, "International Health Policy and Stagnating Maternal Mortality: Is There a Causal Link?" *Reproductive Health Matters* 17, no. 3 (2009): 91–104.

74 Saxena, 2011: 193.

75 This is precisely why Mohan Rao (2005) maintains that the Cairo Conference had negligible benefits for women. He argues that health rights cannot be achieved

under privatized neoliberal developments where the state has retreated from providing health care. The vacuum has been filled by a huge and unregulated private sector that seeks profits at the cost of effective care.

76 Maya Unnithan, "Infertility and Assisted Reproductive Technologies (ARTs) in a Globalising India: Ethics, Medicalisation and Reproductive Agency," *Asian Bioethics Review* 2, no. 1 (2010): 3–18.

77 S. Sharma, S. Mittal, and P. Aggarwal, "Management of Infertility in Low Resource Countries," *International Journal of Obstetrics & Gynaecology* 116, no. 1 (October 2009): 77–83.

78 Widge, 2005. Also Marcia Inhorn, "Reproductive Exile in Global Dubai: South Asian Stories, *Cultural Dynamics* 8, no. 2 (2012): 283–308.

79 Vidya Krishnan, "India's Draft Surrogacy Bill Bars Homosexuals, Live-in Couples," *Live Mint*, August 7, 2013, accessed on March 25, 2014. http://www.livemint.com/Politics/ZsS2zs7KvqHlk4FCguWoEN/Draft-surrogacy-Bill-bars-homosexuals-livein-couples.html.

80 Aarti Dhar, "Gaps in Surrogacy Bill," *Hindu*, October 27, 2013, accessed on March 25, 2014. http://www.thehindu.com/features/metroplus/society/gaps-in-surrogacy-bill/article5276062.ece.

81 Though the Indian Council of Medical Research has a set of guidelines that regulate assisted reproductive technologies, there is no law governing the marketing of these medical interventions. The draft Assisted Reproductive Technology (Regulation) Bill proposed to become law has undergone various revisions, from the 2008 version to the 2010 form to its current 2013 avatar.

82 Shellee Colen (1995), who first used the phrase in 1985, explains that stratified reproduction refers to the "physical and social reproductive tasks [that] are accomplished differentially according to the inequalities that are based on hierarchies of class, race, ethnicity, gender, place in a global economy, and migration status . . . [which are] . . . structured by social, economic, and political forces." Through her classic study of white middle-class New Yorkers who hired West Indian nannies, she reveals how the latter's mothering abilities are both valued and devalued. They are sought out because they are seen as phenomenal caregivers yet the labor they can expend in raising their own children is given short shrift. Various other scholars call these networks of caring relationships that crisscross homes, neighborhoods, class and national borders, care chains. See Arlie Hochschild, "Global Care Chains and Emotional Surplus Value," in Will Hutton and Anthony Giddens, eds., *On the Edge: Living with Global Capitalism* (London: Jonathan Cape, 2000); Rhacel Parreñas, *Servants of Globalization: Women, Migration, and Domestic Work* (Stanford: Stanford University Press, 2001).

83 Mother-work is defined as the unpaid work of reproduction and child rearing. See Molly Ladd-Taylor, *Mother-Work: Women, Child Welfare, and the State, 1890–1930* (Urbana: University of Illinois Press, 1994).

84 I attended a surrogacy "workshop" in Dallas in January 2009. A medical tourism company had brought its in vitro medical specialist from Mumbai to meet with American intended parents in the Hyatt Regency at the Dallas Airport because all attendees, myself included, flew in for the two-hour workshop and flew back to our respective hometowns on the same day.

85 Quoted in Jamie Peck, *Work-Place: The Social Regulation of Labor Markets* (New York: Guilford Press, 1996), 23.

86 Ibid., 24–40.

87 Abigail Haworth, "Surrogate Mothers: Wombs for Rent," *Marie Claire*, July 29, 2007. http://www.marieclaire.com/world-reports/news/international/surrogate-mothers-india. Accessed on July 2, 2009.

Polly Dunbar, "Wombs for Rent: Childless British Couples Pay Indian Women to Carry Their Babies," *MailOnline*, December 8, 2007, accessed on June 20, 2014. http://www.dailymail.co.uk/news/article-500601/Wombs-rent-Childless-British-couples-pay-Indian-women-carry-babies.html. Lisa Fitterman, "Surrogacy in India," *Chatelaine*, March 30, 2009, accessed on June 20, 2014. http://www.chatelaine.com/living/surrogacy-in-india/.

88 Galbraith, McLachlan, and Swales (2005) argue that the largest transaction costs in surrogacy involve surrogate mothers, where intended parents face the task of finding suitable surrogate mothers who may then not complete their contracts and create moral hazards (Galbraith et al., 2005). Incomplete contracts refer to problems that arise when surrogate mothers miscarry, want abortions, or do not want to surrender the newborn. Moral hazards refer to the "post-contractual opportunistic behavior" (Galbraith et al., 2005: 14) exhibited by the surrogate. Once pregnant, she can make financial and nonfinancial/emotional demands on the intended parents, who might feel morally obligated or emotionally blackmailed into meeting her demands. Galbraith et al. (2005: 17–18) say that surrogate mothers too face similar sorts of nonfinancial transaction costs because the intended parents could pay her far less than contracted for once she is pregnant or has delivered the child. Galbraith et al. (2005) maintain that transnational surrogacy agencies can reduce transactional costs to intended parents because these firms take on the responsibility of screening women, enforcing contracts, and controlling "post-contractual opportunistic behavior" that surrogate mothers or intended parents might engage in. See Mhairi Galbraith, Hugh V. McLachlan, and J. Kim Swales, "Commercial Agencies and Surrogate Motherhood: A Transaction Cost Approach," *Health Care Analysis* 11, no. 25 (March 2005): 11–31.

CHAPTER 2. CONVERTING SOCIAL NETWORKS INTO LABOR MARKETS

1 *Punya* is a Kannada word that translates as fortune. A person can have good or bad *punya*. *Punya* is not earned; people are simply fortunate enough to enjoy

advantages or suffer disadvantages that accrue to them because of their past lives. The *punya* one has does not require any effort in this life.

2 Sarita told me she was a flight attendant for Singapore Airlines between the ages of nineteen and twenty-one, which was how she met her alleged boyfriend who was so besotted with her that he named all his various business endeavors after Sarita's daughter. Yet she claimed her relationship with this man was not sexually consummated. She had received her M.A. in English and was a voice trainer for a call center that worked with American and British clients. She had received her M.A. in Dance. She was a lecturer in a college in Bangalore and needed to leave the city on a regular basis because she had to proctor exams or work as an external examiner in smaller towns. She was also getting her MBA.

3 See Loic Wacquant, "Inside the Zone: The Social Art of the Hustler in the Black American Ghetto," *Theory, Culture, and Society* 15, no. 2 (May 1998): 1–36. Also see Sudhir Venkatesh, "'Doin' the Hustle': Constructing the Ethnographer in the American Ghetto," *Ethnography* 3, no. 1 (March 2002): 91–111.

4 In recent long-distance telephone conversations, though, Roopa tells me she has changed her mind. She is currently engaged in a bitter divorce battle in court. Her husband wants her to sign papers in return for the $2,500 he will give as settlement; but Roopa is adamant. She wants him to take on the financial responsibility for raising their daughter or relinquish all paternal rights to the child.

5 My daughter benefited from Roopa's talents in tailoring. She had cut up a silk sari and sewn matching long skirts and blouses for our two girls. "They can look like sisters now," she said smilingly, as she handed me her beautiful gift.

6 Many of the egg donors Roopa enlisted, including her best friend Madhavi, were recent migrants to the city from the northern part of the state. Many worked as construction workers in Bangalore. They were all strong, but small and emaciated women. COTW paid egg donors $500, yet these construction workers received $200 for their eggs which was far below the rates women received for their eggs. Some other doctors, notably Dr. Gunasheela paid egg donors a standard $760 fee for their oocytes. However, recruiting agents such as Suma do not like going there because donors are expected to pay for their screening tests. They lose this money if they do not pass these tests. Also, Dr. Gunasheela refused to pay recruiting agents brokerage fees. Roopa did not have an explanation for the drastic difference in COTW's compensatory practices. In recent conversations Roopa tells me that the number of egg donors being recruited by COTW has ratcheted up exponentially, especially among construction workers in the city. Given the eugenic nature of markets in human eggs, I wondered who purchased these women's eggs. Would they meet commissioning parents' requirements regarding attractiveness, body size, overall health and other such ostensible indicators of fetal and child well-being? Why was COTW recruiting so many egg donors, and why were they paid so little? I wonder if these construction workers' ova are being

channeled toward stem cell experimental technologies? This, however, is a different project altogether.

7 Of these, three older garment workers had been surrogate mothers a decade earlier in a government-run medical facility. These women were not gestational surrogate mothers. Gestational surrogate mothers do not have a genetic relationship to the babies they birth; instead, third-party fertilized eggs are implanted in their bodies.

8 The Kannada word *bele* translates as value or worth. The word's meaning is defined by the context, whether the reference is the cost of onions or the importance of someone's opinions.

9 See Viviana Zelizer, *Purchase of Intimacy* (Princeton: Princeton University Press, 2005): 290–291. She explains that intimate relationships and economic relationships are interrelated through circuits of commerce. She identifies four characteristics to these circuits: First, a circuit has well-defined boundaries and social actors maintain control over goods/ duties/ labor that cross these boundaries. Second, personal interconnections or networks allow the transfer of well-defined goods. Third, some of these transfers involve the use of a specific medium such as money. And fourth, connections between participants are based upon shared meanings.

10 Ibid., 35.

11 Ibid., 298.

12 Jane L. Collins, *Threads: Gender, Labor, and Power in the Global Apparel Industry* (Chicago: University of Chicago Press, 2003), 13. Also see Peck, 1996.

13 Interestingly, most advertising and "infomercial" type programs on surrogacy run on regional language TV channels, that is, Kannada. English and Hindi television programs do not run these programs. My sense is that most working-class individuals in Bangalore watch Kannada programs more often than they watch English or Hindi television. The reproduction industry recruits from working-class communities and it makes economic sense for COTW to target programs popular among working-class communities. A similar trend has been observed in Delhi, where advertisements for surrogacy services are in English but "employees wanted" advertisements are all in Hindi. I thank Namita Kohli for making this observation.

14 James P. Womack, "Just-in-Time Production Systems," in *The Blackwell Encyclopedia of Management*, 2nd edition, ed. Chris Argyris, William Starbuck, and Cary L. Cooper, vol. 5 of *Human Resource Management*, ed. Susan Cartwright (Malden: Blackwell, 2005), 216. Accessed on September 25, 2013.

15 Taken from http://www.toyota-global.com/company/vision_philosophy/toyota_production_system/just-in-time.html. Accessed on September 26, 2013.

16 Peter Stoll, "Three Ethnographies of Escape via Pyramid Schemes," *Anthropological Quarterly* 86, no. 1 (2013): 277–285. The originators of pyramid schemes claim inventory is being depleted rapidly, yet sales may occur only

between people inside the pyramid structure, or through bringing in new recruits into the pyramid rather than reaching out to actual consumers.

17 Ibid., 278.

CHAPTER 3. THE MANY MEANINGS OF SURROGACY

1 I met Mangala because she worked in COTW's front office. She traveled with the agency's egg donors to the neighboring state of Tamil Nadu to Chennai if and when there was a demand for egg donors there. Over subsequent visits to Bangalore I interviewed Mangala too because she had lost her husband to an illness. She needed money, and was considering becoming a surrogate mother herself. She was going to join her younger sister, Geeta, who had miscarried but wanted to try again.

2 I write about Salma in "From Sweatshops to Intimate Labor: Employment Strategies among Surrogate Mothers in Bangalore, India" (translated into French) for a special issue on reproductive technologies in *Les Cahiers du Genre. Biotechonologies et Travail reproducif. Une Perspective Transnationale*, ed. Ilana Lowy, Virginie Rozee, and Lawrence Tain, 56 (2014): 59–86.

3 I write extensively about Indirani in "India's Reproductive Assembly Line," *Contexts* 11, no. 2 (2012): 22–27.

4 Indirani says in Kannada, "*Nijja*, madam. *Makkalu mele nanage yellu ashtu aase illa*." And, she advised her coresidents at the dorm that "*magu mele aase bara kududhu*," or they should not desire to hold onto that baby.

5 As per South Indian kinship rules such alliances are highly desirable. Marriages between women and their maternal cousins (mother's brother's sons) and maternal uncles are seen as good marriages because the bride is received by her matrilineal kin group, which is ostensibly going to embrace her into their extended fold; such acceptance might be more difficult to achieve if she were married to families outside the kin network. The practice of consanguineous marriage is prevalent in all the administrative districts of the south Indian states, Andhra Pradesh, Karnataka, Kerala, and Tamil Nadu. See Allan Holland Bittles, J. Mike Coble, and Naropntul Appaji Rao, "Trends in Consanguineous Marriage in Karnataka, South India, 1980–89," *Journal of Biosocial Sciences* 25, no. 1 (1993): 111–116. Recent demographic research shows that one type of preferred marriage in the Dravidian marriage system—that is, the maternal uncle-niece alliance—is conspicuously absent in Kerala. While the rates of such marriages have not fallen in Karnataka, the states of Tamil Nadu and Andhra Pradesh have seen declines in such marriage alliances. See S. Krishnamoorthy and Narayanaswamy Audinarayana, "Trends in Cosanguinity in South India," *Journal of Biosocial Sciences* 33, no. 2 (2001): 185–197.

6 In many Hindu castes women are not allowed to inherit their father's property; instead the father provides the newly married woman with a dowry, which is directly transferred to the bridegroom's family and is not under the young

woman's control. One way by which these young women can eventually establish their place in the marital family is by producing male offspring. See Bina Agarwal, *A Field of One's Own: Gender and Land Rights in South Asia* (Cambridge: Cambridge University Press, 1994).

7 Arlie Hochschild, *The Managed Heart: The Commercialization of Feeling* (Berkeley: University of California Press, 1983). Also see Arlie Hochschild, *The Commercialization of Intimate Life: Notes from Home and Work* (Berkeley: University of California Press, 2003); Arlie Hochschild, *Outsourced Self: Intimate Life in Market Times* (New York: Metropolitan Books, 2012).

8 Hochschild, 2012: 224.

9 Hochschild, 1983: 85.

10 *Ibid.*, 194.

11 *Ibid.*, 85.

12 Hochschild, 2012: 225.

13 *Ibid.*

14 See Marilyn Strathern, *The Gender of the Gift: Problems with Women and Problems with Society in Melanesia* (Berkeley: University of California Press, 1990), xii.

15 Ibid., 150.

16 Ibid., xi. Marilyn Strathern is making a far more interesting point than the plebian one I am making here; her point is not that women are exchanged. That has already been well established. Instead, she notes that the gift itself is gendered. Thus, the basis of classification of something as a male or female (gift) "does not inhere in the objects themselves but in how they are transacted and to what ends. The action is gendered activity." Strathern continues: "To ask about the gender of the gift, then, is to ask about the situation of gift exchange in relation to the form that domination takes in these societies. It is also to ask about the "gender" of analytical concepts, the worlds that particular assumptions sustain" (1990: xii). But the question remains, What if that "thing" being transacted, say a woman or a child, has subjectivity and an identity that has inhered to "it" prior to "its" status as a gift that is circulated socially?

17 Gayle Rubin, "Traffic in Women: Notes on the 'Political Economy' of Sex," in *Deviations: A Gayle Rubin Reader* (Durham: Duke University Press, 2011), 44.

18 Claude Levi Strauss, *Elementary Structures of Kinship* (Boston: Beacon Press, 1969), 481.

19 Rubin, 2011: 45. Emphasis in original.

20 Given the resurgence of the word "trafficking," almost always used to convey the transfer of women across borders for the purposes of sexual exploitation, Gayle Rubin in a later essay ruefully examines her startling title, taken from Emma Goldman's 1910 essay with the exact same title, "The Traffic in Women" (2011, chapter 2). Just as Goldman did, Rubin says, "The inequalities in gender and class structure respectable institutions such as marriage as much as they (do)

disreputable occupations as prostitution. Putting marriage on an even plane with prostitution highlight(s) how their shared elements, such as the exchange of sex, money, intimacy, or domestic service for room and board reveal(s) much about women's limited choices, poor pay, and marginal power" (2011: 84). To focus exclusively on trafficked women as victims of sexual vice, Rubin notes, is to miss the pervasive, everyday traffic in women. Fixating on sensationalist, moralizing crusades against such "crimes," permits and even endorses muteness on the nonsensational, prosaic matters of everyday injustice. See Gayle Rubin, "The Trouble with Trafficking: Afterthoughts on 'The Traffic in Women,'" in *Deviations: A Gayle Rubin Reader* (Durham: Duke University Press, 2011).

21 Viviana Zelizer, *The Social Meanings of Money* (Princeton: Princeton University Press, 1997).

22 Deniz Kandiyoti, "Bargaining with Patriarchy," *Gender & Society* 2, no. 3 (1988): 275.

CHAPTER 4. LOCATING SURROGACY IN CHILD SHARING AND WAGE LABOR

1 The heavens prophesy that queen Devaki's eighth child will kill her brother Kamsa, the evil king of Mathura. To avoid his fate Kamsa imprisons his sister Devaki and her husband, and kills every child born to them. Devaki is ominously pregnant the eighth time. Her close friend Yashoda who is also pregnant agrees to exchange her newborn daughter for Devaki's newborn son, who is Krishna. Kamsa kills Yashoda's daughter, believing her to be Devaki's offspring. Yashoda raises Krishna as her own child along her with her firstborn son. According to folksongs Krishna later kills his evil uncle king Kamsa for having murdered his baby sister (Kirin Narayan, personal communication). Kirin Narayan, author of *Mondays on the Dark Night of the Moon: Himalayan Foothill Folktales* (Oxford: Oxford University Press, 1997) says that this particular folk story is narrated as a critique of female infanticide practiced in the Himalayan foothills; that is, god will punish those who kill baby girls.

2 Such practices are common elsewhere in the world too, not just in India. Describing West Indian societies, Shellee Colen (1995) notes that stigma is attached to childlessness. Raising more than one generation of children increased women's respect in the larger society. She locates what she calls fostering in this prevailing practice of child care; when mothers left the islands and went to the United States for work, a community of West Indian women took on child care tasks. She explains, "[F]ostering is an extension of the activities, relationships, and values associated with motherhood in West Indian culture. It carries rich meanings and creates webs of interdependent ties in which social and economic resources are shared across time and space through the temporary transferral of parental rights in children. Fostering is central to the experience of migration and reproduction for the West Indian mothers working in New York homes" (1995: 84–85).

3 A fuller version of this section appears in my 2014 article, "From Sweatshops to Intimate Labor: Employment Strategies Among Surrogate Mothers in Bangalore, India," (translated into French).

4 See Meenu Tewari, "Footloose Capital, Intermediation, and the Search for the 'High Road' in Low Wage Industries," in *Labour in Global Production Networks in India*, ed. Anne Posthuma and Dev Nathan (New Delhi: Oxford University Press, 2010), 146–165. Caraway (2007) says that in the start-up phase export-oriented industries tend to be labor intensive and tend to hire women. As industries become more capital intensive, male workers replace their female counterparts. See Teri L. Caraway, *Assembling Women: The Feminization of Global Manufacturing* (Ithaca: Cornell University Press, 2007). There is no evidence to suggest that the Indian garment industry is becoming more capital intensive. Traditionally men and not women have worked as tailors who sewed custom-made clothes for men and women. Hiring practices in garment factories might reflect these earlier trends. No research, though, explains why the southern states of Tamil Nadu and Karnataka hire more women.

5 In 1950 Bangalore had a population of 800,000; of these 28,000 adults worked in textiles. Bangalore Woolen, Cotton and Silk Mills Company Ltd. hired 7,486 workers, the Mysore Spinning and Manufacturing Company Ltd. employed 3,700 workers, and Minerva Mills 3,100 workers. In addition, numerous households operated smaller looms; there were nearly 8,000 looms in the city, with weaving employing 12,990 persons. Other small factories, such as tanning, soap, tobacco, and vegetable oil factories all put together employed just 3,932 persons. See Smriti Srinivas, *Landscapes of Urban Memory: The Sacred and the Civic in India's High Tech City* (Minneapolis: University of Minnesota Press, 2001), 8.

6 Ibid., 10–14.

7 Narendar Pani and Nikky Singh, *The Borders Within: Women, Work, and the Family at the Far End of Globalization* (Bangalore: National Institute for Advanced Studies, n.d.), 14.

8 From their website www.gokaldas.com, accessed on September 22, 2011. Karnataka is one of those Indian states where the garment industry has witnessed rapid growth, with Bangalore being at the center of it all. See D. Rajashekar and Ramachandra Manjula, "Voices of the Women Garment Workers," in *Gender Sensitivity at Workplace*, ed. B. C. Prabhakar (Geneva: ILO, 2006). Just as the government had taken the initiative to build Information Technology Parks where land and electricity are subsidized for companies, it is presently committed to investing in eleven textile parks around the state of Karnataka. The Doddaballapur Integrated Textile Park (DITPL), located in the Bangalore rural district, is targeted to become the nation's most important power loom production centers. This project is expected to spread across 48 acres and will house 75 weaving units and 8 apparel factories owned and operated by private concerns. The "park" will provide employment for 8,000 persons (http://www.karnataka.

com/industry/textiles.html, accessed on September 23, 2011). Though these numbers may seem small in comparison to Gokaldas's operations, its existence points to the state's new interest in garments.

9 *Galli* means street in Hindi.
10 NTUI, an umbrella of independent unions in India, began the Garment and Textile Workers Union (GATWU) in Bangalore in 2006. By 2007 it had built up a membership of over a thousand workers (Tewari, 2010).
11 Pani and Singh, n.d.: 19–35.
12 Tewari, 2010.
13 Pratima Paul Majumdar, *Health Status of the Garment Workers in Bangladesh* (Dhaka: Bangladesh Institute of Development Studies, 2003).
14 Ibid.
15 Melissa Wright, *Disposable Women and Other Myths of Global Capitalism* (New York: Routledge, 2006).
16 Kevin Hewison and Arne L. Kalleberg, "Precarious Work and Flexibilization in South and Southeast Asia," *American Behavioral Scientist* 57, no. 4 (2013): 395–402.
17 First suggested by sociologist C. Wright Mills's *White Collar: The American Middle Class* (New York: Oxford University Press, 1951) and fully developed by Arlie Hochschild in *The Managed Heart* (1983) and Eileen Boris and Rhacel Parreñas in *Intimate Labor* (2010).
18 See Hewison and Kalleberg, 2013: 396.
19 See Chayanika Shah, "Regulate Technology, Not Lives: A Critique of the Draft ART (Regulation) Bill," *Indian Journal of Medical Ethics* 6, no. 1 (2009): 32–35. Also see Imrana Qadeer, "The ART of Marketing Babies," *Indian Journal of Medical Ethics* 7, no. 4 (2010): 209–215.

CHAPTER 5. BABIES AS COMMODITIES

1 Nilanjana Roy, "Protecting the Rights of Surrogate Mothers in India," *New York Times*, October 4, 2011, accessed on July 11, 2014. http://www.nytimes.com/2011/10/05/world/asia/05iht-letter05.html?_r=0.
2 The mothers referred to the clients they worked with as "recipients."
3 See Cecilia Van Hollen, *Birth on the Threshold: Childbirth and Modernity in South India* (Berkeley: University of California Press, 2003). Cecilia van Hollen describes the *cimantam* (Tamil versus the Kannada *srimantha*) as something organized by the woman's parents to satisfy the pregnant woman's desires, cravings, or compulsion. The ritual reveres women for the auspiciousness of their fertility, as *sakti*, "the female generative force of the universe," which is linked to women's reproductive capacities (2003: 77). She explains that the *srimantha* is practiced far more widely than before because of the modern forms of capitalist consumption, becoming "a context in which gifts of not only food but also gold, silk, and modern consumer items (such as kitchen appliances) flowed from the pregnant woman's own parents to her husband's family" (2003: 77).

4 When speaking about love in Kannada, the word "heart" is not used; instead, the word *manasu*, which translates as mind or even soul, is used. Kala says in Kannada, "*manasu gatti made aa magu kodu thane*," which I translate as "I will harden my soul and give up that baby." My translation of the interview transcript is not literal here but is an attempt at fidelity of meaning.

5 The word *himse* is a Sanskrit derivative that means harm, injury, violence, or suffering. For example, the directive *himse koda beda* translates as "Do not trouble me." Thus, a person bothering or annoying another is seen as causing harm.

6 To reconfirm that intended parents were indeed being billed, I emailed Elvia with whom I maintain a regular correspondence over email. She replied, "Hi Sharmila, you are correct. The majority of doctors do not give you second chances for free. . . . We had to pay up front for 2 negatives. . . . I bet doctors all over India do not pay the surrogate if they miscarry because it is difficult to get the truth from them" (pers. comm., July 18, 2012).

7 In a subsequent email Elvia wrote, "[D]octors screwing intended parents as well as surrogates is totally the [industry's] untold secret" (pers. comm., July 18, 2012).

8 See Paula England, "Gender Inequality in Labor Markets: The Role of Motherhood and Segregation," *Social Politics* 12, no. 2, 2005: 277.

9 Ibid., 278.

10 Debora Spar, *The Baby Business: How Science, Money, and Politics Drive the Commerce of Conception* (Boston: Harvard Business School Press, 2006); Naomi Cahn, *Test Tube Families: Why The Fertility Market Needs Legal Regulation* (New York: NYU Press, 2009); Amrita Pande, "Commercial Surrogacy in India: Manufacturing a Perfect Mother-Worker," *Signs* 35, no. 4 (2010): 969–992.

11 Spar, 2006: xi.

12 Ibid., 207.

13 Ibid., 195.

14 Ibid., 197.

15 Cahn, 2009: 235.

16 Pande, 2010.

17 Spar, 2006: 207.

18 Ibid., 209.

19 Bhalla and Thapliyal, 2013; Hillary Brenhouse, "India's Rent-a-Womb Industry Faces New Restrictions," *Time*, June 5, 2010, accessed April 2, 2014. http://content.time.com/time/world/article/0,8599,1993665,00.html. Scott Carney, "Inside India's Rent-a-Womb Business," *Mother Jones*, March/April 2010, accessed April 11, 2014. http://www.motherjones.com/politics/2010/02/surrogacy-tourism-india-nayna-patel; *Daily Mail* Reporter, "The Baby Factory: In a Huge Clinic in India, Hundreds of Women Are Paid £5,000 Each to Have Western Couples' Babies," *Daily Mail Online*, October 1, 2013, accessed on April 2, 2014. http://www.dailymail.co.uk/news/ article-2439977/The-baby-factory-In-huge-clinic-India-hundreds-women-paid-5–000-Western-couples-babies.html; Sam Dolnick,

"India's Baby Farm," *Sunday Morning Herald*, January 6, 2008, accessed July 25, 2012. http://www.smh. com.au/ news/world/indias-baby-farm/2008/01/05/1198950126650.html?page=fullpage#contentSwap2. Haworth, 2007; Gayatri Jayaraman, "The Baby Factory: Surrogacy, the Booming Business in Gujarat," *India Today*, August 23, 2013, accessed April 2, 2014. http://indiatoday.intoday.in/story/surrogacy-blooming-business-in-gujarat-shah-rukh-aamir-khan/1/301026.htm; Sandra Schulz, "The Life Factory: In India, Surrogacy Has Become a Global Business," *Spiegel Online International*, September 25, 2008, accessed April 2, 2014. http://www.spiegel.de/international/world/0,1518,580209-2,00.html. Adrianne Vogt, "The Rent-a-Womb Boom," *The Daily Beast*, March 1, 2014, accessed April 2, 2014. http://www.thedailybeast.com/witw/articles/2014/03/01/the-rent-a-womb-boom-is-india-s-surrogacy-industry-empowering-or-exploitative.html.

20 *Sambla* is wages and *badige* is rent.

21 Marx writes, "[W]hat distinguishes the worst architect from the best of bees is this, that the architect raises his structure in imagination before he erects it in reality. At the end of every labor process, we get a result that already existed in the imagination of the laborer at its commencement." Thus, an architect's creativity, intellect, emotions, and individual will shape the eventual product she creates. And, the product has history. Whereas a bee has no individual will—only pure instinct—in making that hive which has no history. Karl Marx, "Capital, Volume One," in *The Marx-Engels Reader*, 2nd edition, ed. Robert C. Tucker (New York: W. W. Norton, 1978), 334–345.

22 Mary O'Brien, *The Politics of Reproduction* (Boston: Routledge & Kegan Paul, 1981), 38.

23 Nancy Hartsock, *The Feminist Standpoint Revisited and Other Essays* (Boulder: Westview Press, 1998).

24 Micaela di Leonardo introduces the term "kin work" to describe such reciprocity by which she means:

> the conception, maintenance, and ritual celebration of cross-household kin ties, including visits, letters, telephone calls, presents, and cards to kin; the organization of holiday gatherings; the creation and maintenance of quasi-kin relations; decisions to neglect or to intensify particular ties; the mental work of reflection about all these activities; and the creation and communication of altering images of family and kin vis-à-vis the images of others, both folk and mass media (1987: 442–443).

Di Leonardo introduces "kin work" because she wants to highlight all the emotion work women engage in that does not count as household or domestic labor but is a crucial means of maintaining social ties with kin groups (fictive or otherwise). Women, more than men, perform kin work. Micaela di Leonardo, "The Female World of Cards and Holidays: Women, Families, and the Work of Kinship," *Signs* 12, no. 3 (Spring 1987): 440–453.

25 Chandra used the word *sank-ta*, which translates as torment or anguish. For many mothers to be alone and apart from family is anguish.

26 The few times I have presented this topic in conferences and other public fora, audience members have been horrified at the idea of multiple embryo transplants and fetal reduction. However, research shows that multiple embryo transfers are also the norm in the United States. Single embryonic rates were highest in Sweden (69.4 percent) but are as low as 2.8 percent in the United States, indicating that fetal reductions in IVF procedures are perhaps just as common here as they are in India. See Abha Maheshwari, Siriol Griffiths, and Siladitya Bhattacharya, "Global Variations in the Uptake of Single Embryo Transfer," *Human Reproduction Update* 12, no. 1 (2011): 107–120.

27 Amrita Pande documents how one mother, Parvati, felt about fetal reduction:

> Doctor Madam told us that the babies wouldn't get enough space to move around and grow, so we should get the surgery. But both Nandinididi [the genetic mother] and I wanted to keep all three. We had informally decided on that. I told Doctor Madam that I'll keep one and didi can keep two. After all it's my blood even if it's their genes. And who knows whether at my age I'll be able to have more babies.

Amrita Pande, "'It May be Her Eggs But It's My Blood': Surrogates and Everyday Forms of Kinship in India," *Qualitative Sociology* 32, no. 4 (2009): 379–397.

28 Amrita Pande reveals something similar in her work, when she quotes one mother as saying the following:

> See, with your husband's child there is a constant relation, every night there is a "process" [she makes a gesture with her hands to show penetration] and this makes the child grow. The small seed swells up like this [she mimics a balloon being inflated by a pump] and in nine months is ready to be out. But with surrogacy there is no contact with either your husband or the other male [the biological father] so the child has to be grown by giving me injections (2009: 385).

29 In colloquial Kannada, *udhara* refers to good fortune.

30 Simmel, 51.Whereas Marx holds that the value of an object is determined by the socially useful labor needed to produce it, the notion of sacrifice looms large in Georg Simmel's theory of exchange. Georg Simmel, *On Individuality and Social Forms*, ed. Donald N. Levine (Chicago: Chicago University Press, 1971).

31 Simmel says, "[A]ll labor is indisputably a sacrifice if it is accompanied by a desire for leisure, for the mere self-satisfying play of skills, or for the avoidance of strenuous exertion (Simmel, 1971: 49). Marx would concur that labor effort is absolute sacrifice when he observes:

> [L]abor is *external* to the laborer—that is, it is not part of his nature—and that the worker does not affirm himself in his work but denies himself, feels miserable and unhappy, develops no free physical and mental energy but

mortifies his flesh and ruins his mind. The worker . . . feels at ease only outside work, and during work he is outside himself. He is at home when he is not working and when he is working he is not at home. His work, therefore, is not voluntary but coerced, *forced labor*. It is not the satisfaction of a need, but only a *means* to satisfy other needs. Its alien character is obvious from the fact that as soon as no physical or other pressure exists, labor is avoided like the plague. External labor, labor in which man is externalized, is the labor of self-sacrifice, of penance (1994: 61–62. Emphasis in original). *Karl Marx: Selected Writings*, ed. Lawrence Simon (Indianapolis: Hackett, 1994).

32 See Simmel 1971: 49–50. He explains: "[F]or this quantum of energy there compete a number of demands all of which it cannot satisfy. For every expenditure of the energy in question one or more possible and desirable alternative uses of it must be sacrificed. Could we not usefully spend the energy with which we accomplish task A also on task B, then the first would not entail any sacrifice; the same would hold for B in the event we chose it rather than A. In this utilitarian loss what is sacrificed is not labor, but *non-labor*. What we pay for A is not the sacrifice of labor—for our assumption here is that the latter in itself poses not the slightest hardship on us—but the giving up of task B" (1971: 49).

33 Pushpa was not a garment worker; instead, she was employed as a cook. She was also the only woman I interviewed who did not belong to the networks of mothers I had been in conversation with. She had got to know Suma during her stay in COTW and through this friendship, came to meet me and be interviewed. We met three times over the summer of 2011. I do not know whether she faces infertility because of her ectopic pregnancy, which required hospitalization.

34 The Center for Disease Control provides statistics for various American infertility clinics on their website; the CDC notes that the 30–35 percent of the IVF cycles result in live births for women under the age of 35. Thus, 65–70 percent of the IVF attempts do not result in live births. The live birth rates through IVF fall as women age. Live birth rates are 25 percent for women between 35–37 years of age; 15–25 percent for women between the ages of 38 to 40, and 6–10 percent for women over the age of 40. http://americanpregnancy.org/infertility/ivf.html. Accessed March 24, 2014. Arguably, surrogacy agencies in India have a better success rate because the women they recruit into the industry are of prime reproductive age.

CHAPTER 6. FETUSES AS PERSONS, SURROGATE MOTHERS AS NONPERSONS

1 Parts of this section are in my article titled "What to Expect When You're Expecting: Consuming Parenthood through Surrogacy in India," (Rudrappa, 2016). The parts on gay fathers appears in "Conceiving Fatherhood: Gay Fathers and Indian Surrogate Mothers," (Rudrappa, 2015).

2 To be sure, gay fathers and straight mothers/fathers relate differently to surrogate mothers' pregnancies. Elsewhere I explain that intended gay fathers are not so different from many heterosexual men who, upon learning about their partners' pregnancies, will similarly announce that "they" are pregnant, rather than seeing it as her exclusive physical/ emotional condition. A woman's pregnancy, because of her bodily, and often, emotional/ intellectual, involvement with the fetus, allows her a kind of closeness and experiential knowledge of the forthcoming child that is not available to men. The fathers may have contributed biologically to the existence of that fetus but the only way they can relate to it is through vicarious visualization. Through imagination, cognition, and love, fathers can potentially grasp at pregnancy. Part of exerting that love for their pregnant partners and the forthcoming child is expressed in these fathers' claim, "we're pregnant." Gay men working with surrogate mothers, however, are different. They do not have a sense of connection with the surrogate mothers as straight men who make such claims when their women partners are pregnant with "their" children. See Rudrappa, "Conceiving Fatherhood," 2015.

3 Janelle Taylor (2004) makes a parallel argument in her work on pregnant straight women, where she notes that the fetus becomes a commodity for the women; commodification, she notes, "is inextricably bound up with personification" (2004: 409). Janelle Taylor, "A Fetish Is Born: Sonographers and the Making of the Public Fetus," in *Consuming Motherhood*, ed. Janelle Taylor, Linda Layne, and Danielle Wozniak (New Brunswick: Rutgers University Press, 2004): 187–210.

4 This aspect of legality did not come up in my interviews, and I thank Sam Everingham for this invaluable insight. Given his advocacy for Australian straight and gay parents who might need surrogacy services, I felt it was appropriate to share with him an article I had written earlier on gay parents in the United States and Australia. Mr. Everingham says that through his work he has met innumerable individuals who were unsure about their status regarding the surrogated baby. In some cases in Australia, he says, fathers with a genetic relation to the surrogated babies—*their* babies who they are raising in deeply committed ways—are legally recognized as only "sperm donors," and not fathers.

5 For example, Jason Hanna and Joe Riggs, a Texas gay couple, were denied the fatherhood of two boys born through domestic surrogacy even though the babies were genetically descended from them. As of 2015, in Texas surrogacy contracts are legal between a married couple and an agency; but, same-sex marriages are not legally recognized in the state and any surrogacy contract a gay couple may enter into is not accorded legal recognition. Therefore the Dallas judge concluded that Hanna and Riggs's surrogacy contract was invalid, and on the birth certificate only the name of the surrogate mother, who has no genetic relationship to the babies, was listed. The twins were in the custody of the two gay fathers who provided them with their daily care, but they were not legal fathers to their own sons. Kristy Watkins, "Unpredictable Laws or Discrimination?" *Gender & Society*,

July 14, 2014, accessed on January 12, 2015. https://gendersociety.wordpress.com/2014/07/14/unpredictable-laws-or-discrimination/.

6 Elvia is not alone in her quest for racial matching. One of the mothers I met went so far as to pay her cousin for her eggs. The cousin traveled to India to have her ova extracted in order to facilitate the pregnancy. It was important for the intended mother to enhance the chances of having blonde children who would look like her. Various other scholars observe that intended mothers who use an egg donor's services attempt to enhance perceived genetic closeness. Becker, Butler, and Nachtigall (2005) note that this issue arose as well among gamete donor families they'd interviewed. That is, the lack of familial resemblance can be a source of significant anxiety for parents when they are with their children in public. See Gay Becker, Anneliese Butler, and Robert D. Nachtigall, "Resemblance Talk: A Challenge for Parents Whose Children Were Conceived with Donor Gametes in the U.S.," *Social Science and Medicine* 61, No. 6 (2005): 1300–1309.

7 Petchesky writes:

> Women's responses to fetal picture taking may have another side as well, rooted in their traditional role in the production of family photographs. If photographs accommodate "aesthetic consumerism," becoming instruments of appropriation and possession, this is nowhere truer than within family life—particularly middle-class family life. Family albums originated to chronicle the continuity of Victorian bourgeois kin networks. The advent of home movies in the 1940s and 1950s paralleled the move to the suburbs and backyard barbeques. Similarly, the presentation of a sonogram photo to the dying grandfather, even before his grandchild's birth, is a 1980s way of affirming patriarchal lineage. In other words, far from the intrusion of an alien, and alienating, technology, it may be that ultrasonography is becoming enmeshed in a familiar language of "private" images (1987: 283).

Rosalind Petchesky, "Fetal Images: The Power of Visual Culture in the Politics of Reproduction," *Feminist Studies* 12, no. 2 (1987): 263–292. Also see Janelle Taylor's monograph, *The Public Life of the Fetal Sonogram: Technology, Consumption, and the Politics of Reproduction* (New Brunswick: Rutgers University Press, 2008).

8 See Janelle Taylor, "Of Sonograms and Baby Prams: Fetal Diagnosis, Pregnancy, and Consumption," *Feminist Studies* 26, no. 2 (2000): 401.

9 Ibid., 403.

10 Elly Teman, *Birthing a Mother: The Surrogate Body and the Pregnant Self* (Berkeley: University of California Press, 2010).

11 All the names have been changed. *Gudia* means doll; *Sona* means gold, or precious; and *rani* means queen in Hindi.

12 The relationships between clients and surrogate mothers were much like Georg Simmel describes regarding relationships mediated by money: Money, he writes, "is never an adequate means in a relationship between persons that depends on

duration and integrity. . . . Money serves most matter-of-factly and completely for venal pleasure, which rejects any continuation of the relationship beyond sensual satisfaction. . . . When one pays money one is completely quits." Simmel, 1971: 121.

13 Melissa Wright says that myths' "usefulness derives largely from their claims to unquestionable authority" (2006: 3). Building from Ronald Barthes, she says that myths empty reality of history. Politics is masked by "narratives of human essence and naturalized tautologies. In consequence, myths are vehicles for foreclosing discussions of politics as they use fantastic characters and situations to depict hierarchical relationships as broadly believed to have bearing on 'real life' without having to explain these relationships" (2006: 3–4). Quoting Talal Asad, Wright continues that myth is "not merely a (mis)representation of the *real*. It [is] material for shaping the possibilities and limits of action" (Asad, 2003, 29, quoted in Wright, 2006: 4).

CHAPTER 7. SURROGACY AS A GIFT

1 Adrienne Arieff, interview with Emanuella Grinberg, "The Highs and Lows of Foreign Surrogacy," *CNN*, March 29, 2012, accessed on July 13, 2014. http://www.cnn.com/2012/03/29/living/sacred-thread-foreign-surrogacy/.

2 Adrienne Arieff, in http://leanin.org/stories/adrienne-arieff/. Accessed on July 11, 2014. Emphasis added. Her book is titled *The Sacred Thread: A True Story of Becoming a Mother and Finding a Family—Half a World Away* (New York: Random House, Inc., 2012).

3 Quoted in "India's Baby Farm," *Sunday Morning Herald*, January 6, 2008, accessed on July 25, 2012. http://www.smh.com.au/news/world/indias-baby-farm/2008/01/05/1198950126650.html?page=fullpage#contentSwap2.

4 Quoted in her interview with Grinberg, 2012.

5 See Amrita Pande, 2011. To read more on "rescue fantasies" regarding adopted children see Laura Briggs, *Somebody's Children: The Politics of Transracial and Transnational Adoption* (Durham: Duke University Press, 2012).

6 Quoted in Brenhouse, 2010.

7 See Muhammad Yunus, "Nobel Lecture," *Nobelprize.org*, December 10, 2006, accessed on January 20, 2015. http://www.nobelprize.org/nobel_prizes/peace/laureates/2006/yunus-lecture-en.html. What Dr. Yunus does not say is that these poor women pay interest rates of close to 24 percent on their small loans. See David Roodman, "Quick: What's the Grameen Bank's Interest Rate?" *Center for Global Development*, September 24, 2010, accessed April 3, 2014. http://www.cgdev.org/blog/quick-whats-grameen-banks-interest-rate.

8 Because of her national prominence in infertility assistance, in 2005 she had served on the Indian Council for Research (ICMR) committee that drafted the National Guidelines for Accreditation, Supervision & Regulation of ART Clinics in India.

9 See Grinberg, 2012.

10 Quoted in Brenhouse, 2010.

11 The commonly used colorful Kannada phrase was "*thalle alle muru kaas saman illa*."
12 I frequently traveled by auto rickshaw in Bangalore. Over these rides I conversed with the drivers who informed me that they were not allowed into the newly constructed Bangalore airport, which affected their ability to get good fares. Also, the newly constructed metro lines, which provide excellent public transportation, contributed to Bangaloreans' decreased dependence on auto rickshaws for transportation.
13 Galbraith et al., 2005: 14.
14 *Atma* refers to soul, consciousness, or the self. *Trupti* loosely translates as satisfaction or the satiation of desire. When the two words are used together, as *atma trupti*, the term refers to satisfaction in the soul, contentment with self, or inner contentment.
15 *Hettha thai* is birth mother.

CONCLUSION

1 Susan Bordo, *Unbearable Weight: Feminism, Western Culture, and the Body* (Berkeley: University of California Press, 1993). Especially important is her chapter, "Are Mothers Persons?"
2 Alison Bailey, "Reconceiving Surrogacy: Toward a Reproductive Justice Account of Indian Surrogacy," *Hypatia* 26, no. 4 (Fall 2011): 715–741.
3 I take this term from Stanley Cohen's *States of Denial: Knowing About Atrocities and Suffering* (Cambridge: Polity Press, 2001). He examines the personal and political ways by which everyday violence is denied by perpetrators and witnesses. I use his work to think through how victims themselves engage in denial; people are in constant denial about the abysmal conditions of their lives. To acknowledge everyday struggles can be immobilizing. Thus, writes Cohen, "moderately depressed people may seem more pessimistic, but their clinical profile shows *less* cognitive distortion than in normal people. Far from distorting reality, they see it only too clearly. They also have a more balanced view of themselves, the world, and their future. Unable to sustain 'positive illusions,' they are doomed to a state of depressive realism. They lack the biases that normally shelter people from the harsher side of reality" (Cohen, 2001: 56).
4 Dorothy Roberts, "Punishing Drug Addicts Who Have Babies: Women of Color, Equality, and the Right to Privacy," *Harvard Law Review* 104 (May 1991): 1436.
5 Ibid., 1455.
6 Krittivas Mukherjee, "The Chhattisgarh Lesson: Cash-for-Sterilisation Drive May Be Masking Grave Tragedy," *Hindustan Times*, November 11, 2014, accessed on January 24, 2015. http://www.hindustantimes.com/comment/analysis/india-s-cash-for-sterilisation-campaign-maybe-masking-a-grave-human-tragedy/article1-1284927.aspx.
7 Rosalinda Pineda Orfeneo, "Economic and Reproductive Justice in the Context of Women in the Informal Economy," *Asian Bioethics Review* 2, no. 1 (2010): 19–35.

INDEX

ABOUT THE AUTHOR

Sharmila Rudrappa is Associate Professor of Sociology and core faculty at the Center for Women's and Gender Studies at the University of Texas at Austin. She also serves as the Director of the Center for Asian American Studies. Her previous publications include *Ethnic Routes to Becoming American: Indian Immigrants and the Cultures of Citizenship*.